ProgressionSeries

Sports Science and Physiotherapy

For entry to university and college in 2010

PUBLISHED BY: UCAS ROSEHILL NEW BARN LANE CHELTENHAM GL52 3LZ

PRODUCED IN CONJUNCTION WITH GTI SPECIALIST PUBLISHERS

© UCAS 2009

ISBN: 978-1-84361-118-9

UCA3 REFERENCE NUMBER: PU040010
PUBLICATION REFERENCE: 09_032

FURTHER COPIES AVAILABLE FROM WWW.UCASBOOKS.COM

POST: UCAS MEDIA PO BOX 130 CHELTENHAM GL52 3ZF
E: publicationservices@ucas.ac.uk   F: +44 (0)1242 544 806

FURTHER INFORMATION ABOUT THE UCAS APPLICATION PROCESS
T: +44 (0)871 468 0 468   F: +44 (0)1242 544 961

CALLS TO THE 0871 NUMBER QUOTED ABOVE FROM BT LANDLINES WITHIN THE UK WILL COST NO MORE THAN £0.09 PER MINUTE.
THE COST OF CALLS FROM MOBILES AND OTHER NETWORKS MAY VARY.

UCAS QUALITY AWARDS

UCAS *gti*

Foreword

THINKING ABOUT SPORTS SCIENCE AND PHYSIOTHERAPY?

Researching the type of course you would like to study at higher education level means that you are halfway towards choosing the right qualification for you. Knowing which subject or subjects you would enjoy is a distinct advantage, but each course can vary depending on the specific areas covered and the university or college you choose to attend. Even if the course title is the same at a number of institutions, it does not mean that the content or teaching methods will be the same. Finding a university or college that will suit you academically and personally can take time.

Throughout the year, there are opportunities to visit different universities and colleges, where advisers can tell you about the courses in detail and you can see where you will be living and studying for the next few years of your life.

Speaking to former students of the course you would like to study is extremely useful – they can give you an insider's view of university life and the teaching standards that you could not find anywhere else. We at UCAS have teamed up with GTI Specialist Publishers to provide careers advice and real-life case studies in *Progression to Sports Science and Physiotherapy*. You will find information on careers in sports science and physiotherapy, how to study these subjects, entry routes, advice on applying through UCAS, and course listings. We hope you find this publication helps you to choose a course and university that are right for you.

Applying for higher education through **www.ucas.com** has never been easier: the UCAS website supplies everything you need to know, from available courses and entry requirements to information on financial help and accommodation. The online application is clear and simple to complete, but help is at hand online or from our team of telephone advisers should you need it.

On behalf of UCAS and GTI Specialist Publishers, I wish you every success in your research.

Anthony McClaran, Chief Executive, UCAS

Introducing sports science and physiotherapy

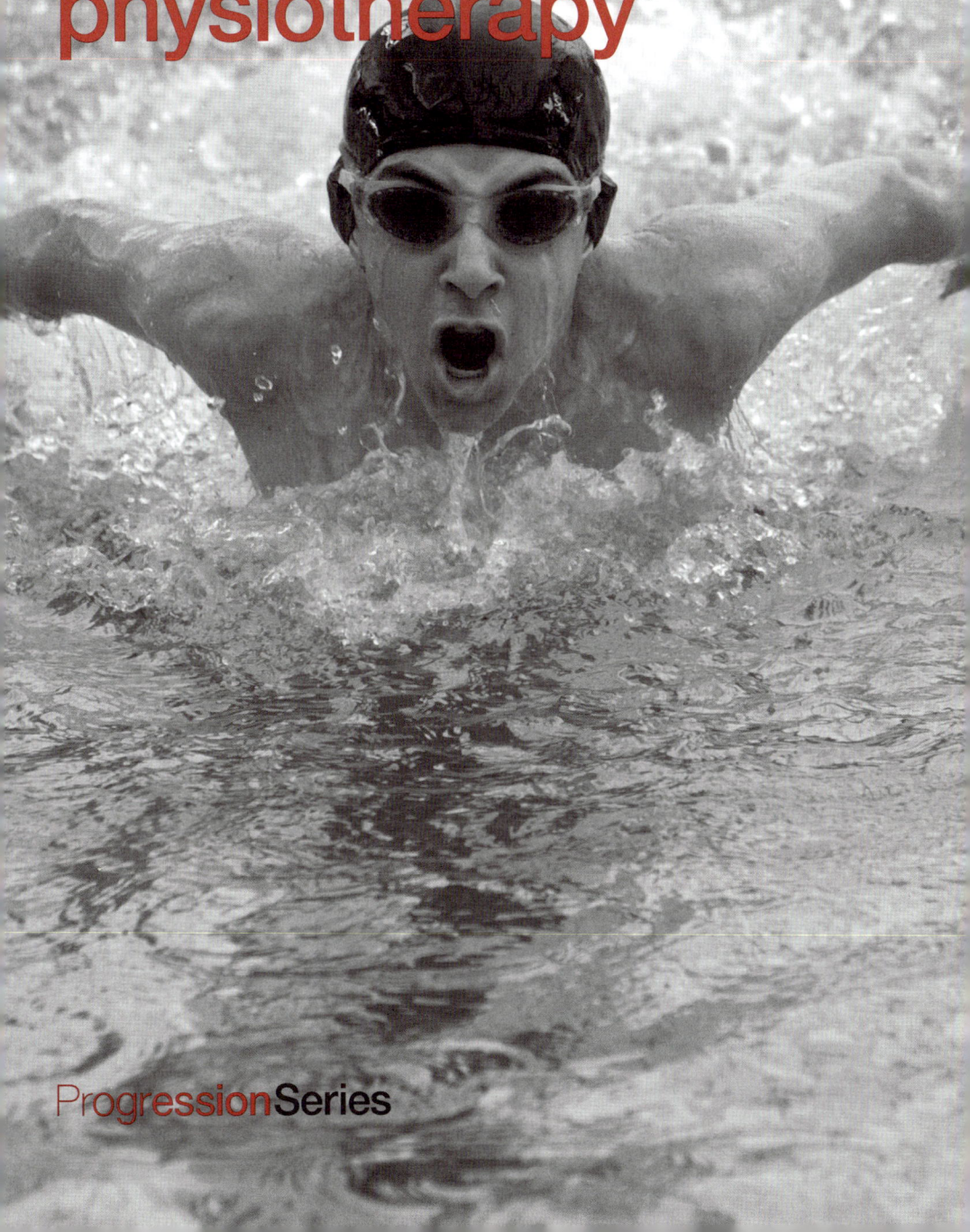

ProgressionSeries

It could be you…

… assessing a swimmer's movement to improve competition timings	– biomechanist
… designing a campaign to encourage people to be more active	– health promotion specialist
… training a football team to win the FA Cup	– sports coach
… advising clients on adapting to normal life after illness or injury	– occupational therapist
… supporting a client to become mobile again after surgery	– physiotherapist
… helping an athlete prepare mentally for competition	– sports psychologist

… and lots more besides. Working in the sports science and physiotherapy fields gives graduates a huge range of choice. From encouraging children from disadvantaged backgrounds to take part in sports to enabling a world-class athlete win the Olympics, you will be making a difference, no matter at what level you practise. Could a career in a sports science-related field be for you?

A CAREERS IN SPORTS SCIENCE AND PHYSIOTHERAPY

A sports coach supporting athletes at international level can earn in excess of £100,000 per year before tax – see **A career in sports science and physiotherapy**, starting on page 13.

As well as any commitment to sports and other physical activities, admissions tutors also look for academic ability, people skills, an analytical approach and a commitment to work hard – see **The career for you?** on page 37.

Getting onto a sports-related degree course isn't a doddle. To see what you need to succeed, read **Routes to qualification** on page 57.

SPORTS SCIENCE AND PHYSIOTHERAPY IN CONTEXT

The reason why sports science and physiotherapy are so popular is because they play a major role in helping a wide variety of people lead more active and successful lives. While this can at one end involve training an athlete to win an Olympic gold, it can also be just as rewarding helping an elderly person learn to walk again after a major stroke. Being active makes a huge difference to people's lives. Think about when you have been either injured or ill and confined to bed. The novelty probably wore off pretty quickly and you wished you were up and about, cycling with your friends or playing football after school, or just walking to the shops. Human beings were made to be mobile and when we're not, our physical and mental health can suffer.

People employed within the sports science and physiotherapy fields use the knowledge and skills that they have gained from their studies and work experience to help people deal with a wide variety of problems. For example, in any one day individuals in this area might be involved in any of the following situations (and plenty more besides):

- enabling a depressed person to get out of the house to enjoy a hobby and meet new people
- coming up with the most effective way to convey a public health message about the negative side effects of unhealthy eating
- restoring a person's feet to a much better condition, thus enabling them to walk more comfortably
- filming and assessing the way in which a runner sprints to see how they can run even faster by adjusting their stride
- counselling an athlete on how to cope with stress in major competitions.

YOUR PART IN SPORTS SCIENCE AND PHYSIOTHERAPY

Are you good with people? Do you have well-honed observation skills and an analytical nature? Great! Because you will need a wide and varied skills set to work in these fields. Many people forget that sports science and physiotherapy are *scientific* in nature, involving the study of such subjects as anatomy, biology, physiology, biomechanics, physics, and even engineering. It's not just about being good at kicking a ball, it's about understanding how kicking it in a certain way might score the winning goal, or how positive thinking might just give someone the confidence to believe they can do it. This is what makes these areas so interesting to work in: they combine personal skills such as listening and observation with very scientific approaches to gathering information to give you the whole picture of what's going on with an athlete – mentally and physically.

If you're interested in a possible career in any of these areas, then this guide can help point you in the right direction. Read on to discover:

- the main areas of work and roles on offer
- what it takes to work in sports science-related areas and physiotherapy
- how to get in and the paths to qualification
- advice from recent graduates on how they got to where they are today.

Why sports science and physiotherapy?

Choose a career that is...

VARIED

There are few careers that offer as much variety as sports science and physiotherapy, in terms of both the people you will deal with and the problems that they face. Leading a more active life is something that everyone needs to aspire to, for their emotional and physical well-being, so being involved in ways that enable them to enjoy exercise and to do it to the best of their ability can be incredibly rewarding. You could be coaching school football teams, teaching dance or aerobics to the elderly or helping a talented long-jumper to adapt their style to become more aerodynamic. Or you could be helping individuals recover from serious illnesses and injuries and giving them hope by assisting them in becoming more mobile. Whatever you do, the buzz you get from helping a person achieve their goals – no matter how big or small – can be amazing.

VITAL TO SOCIETY

While being healthy and active might not be absolutely essential for society to survive, it is certainly becoming such an issue that the government is always looking into new ways to make people more responsible for their lives. This includes changing unhealthy and potentially dangerous eating habits and making the prospect of physical activity more fun. Professionals involved in sports science and physiotherapy are at the forefront of this agenda, advising the general public and other healthcare professionals on how to make small but significant changes that could really turn someone's life around.

TECHNICAL *AND* PEOPLE-FOCUSED

Some careers are so appealing because they offer the chance to use two different types of skills – the opportunity to use your technical or scientific expertise alongside the chance to work with people. In sports science-related areas and physiotherapy, you will definitely be required to do this and therefore you will need a balance and interest in both. You'll use the latest research and technology, but you'll also see how these affect real people – **your** clients.

BECOMING INCREASINGLY IMPORTANT

With the London 2012 Olympics on the horizon, it is estimated that government expenditure in sports science and related areas will increase, bringing with it further career opportunities. As society becomes more aware of the importance of physical activity you could be in the driving seat, alerting people to possibilities, supporting them in becoming involved, looking at ways to make their performance better and helping them if injury strikes.

ALWAYS IN DEMAND

People of all ages and from all walks of life will always need rehabilitative help so your skills, knowledge and expertise will never be out of demand. Additionally, sports are very popular both to watch and to participate in, so there will always be a need for professionals who can help sportsmen and women to achieve their best and recover quickly from injuries. The growing concern over educating people to adopt healthier lifestyles and to teach them good eating habits means that the professionals working in sports science-related areas and physiotherapy will have skills that have never been so valuable as they are today.

WHAT DO SPORTS SCIENCE PROFESSIONALS SAY?

'I enjoy my job because it allows to me to spend all day with a wide variety of people, both fellow medical professionals and patients. It gives me huge satisfaction to see the achievements patients make.'
Jennifer Riley, junior physiotherapist
'I really enjoy educating the students about various aspects of sports psychology, and making them think about their own sporting achievements and how psychology has helped them.'
Jenny Page, senior lecturer in sport and exercise psychology

GET
thinking about
your career

The 2010 GET directory has a new look and new content with more careers advice from experts and recent graduates as well as hundreds of employers

Jobs, courses and advice from the heart

Official travel partner
STA TRAVEL
www.statravel.co.uk

In association with

Sponsored by
PRICEWATERHOUSECOOPERS

get.

50 great careers that
welcome all disciplines

20 tips for perfect applications
20 tricks for interview success

10 types of further study
that look good on a CV

2010

- THE comprehensive graduate careers directory covering every degree discipline and industry sector with EVERY major employer in the UK listed.
- Offering advice, vacancies, company profiles and case studies from recent graduates.
- New for this edition, a postgraduate section offering guidance and an A-Z listing of all institutions offering postgraduate courses in 2010.
- Best of all, it is still FREE to all students from your Careers Service.

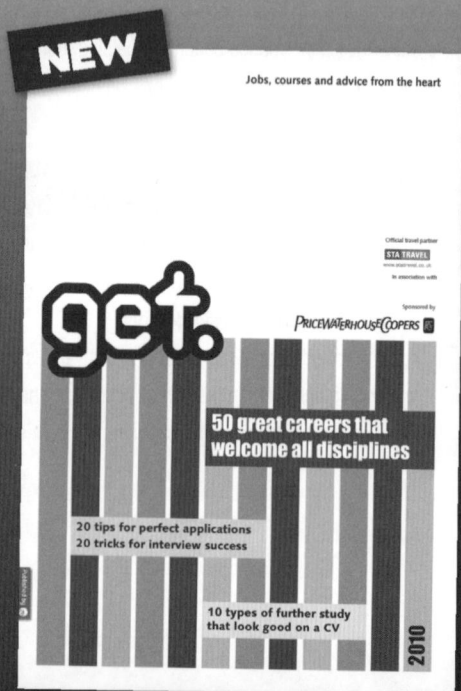

gti media

A career in sports science and physiotherapy

A career in sports science and physiotherapy

Areas of work

This section aims to give you an overview of the main career choices, specialisms, working conditions and pay for those working in sports science and physiotherapy in the UK today.

If you have an interest in both sports and sciences, and a desire to work with people, then a career in sports science and physiotherapy could be for you. At this stage, you don't need to decide on a particular specialty, although you will normally need to make your mind up between a more general sports science degree and the more specific physiotherapy, psychology or podiatry courses, as the training is different between the three and it's not really possible to move from one to the other without starting again in the relevant undergraduate study.

Equally, if you think your interest lies in the very specialised field of sports and exercise psychology, your training route will probably be longer than that undertaken in other fields. This would involve either an undergraduate degree in psychology followed by further postgraduate specialised study in sports psychology, or you could study sports science (or another subject) and then take a psychology conversion course, followed by the relevant postgraduate training.

TIME WELL SPENT

It might seem bewildering to have to make such big decisions now. This is why we have compiled the next section for you, where we look at various job roles within sports science, podiatry, physiotherapy and sports and exercise psychology so you can gain a clearer picture about what's involved in each, including typical responsibilities, working hours, skills required and how much you'll get paid. We also look at the pros and cons and where you can find more information should you choose to investigate further. It is worthwhile spending some time considering your options at this stage so that when you are making your university applications you will know, with confidence, that you have chosen your subject wisely.

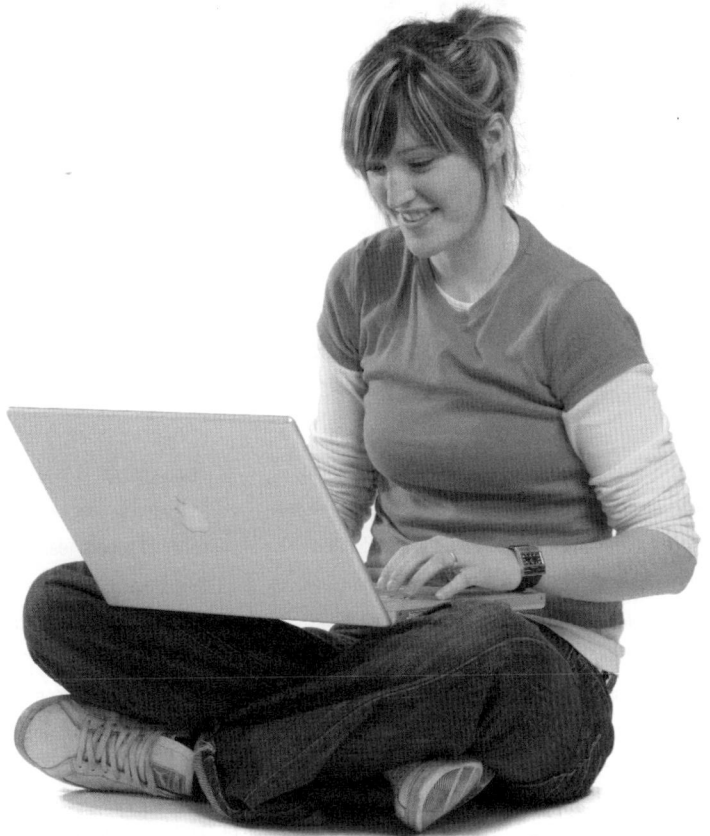

Which area?

Biomechanist

THE WORK

Biomechanics is a very scientific field, covering such diverse aspects as physics, mechanics, biology, mathematics, statistics and anatomy. While it is employed frequently in the sports arena, it is not, in itself, a sports discipline. Rather, biomechanists work with sportsmen and women in an analytical way, to help improve their performance through a scientific study of how certain forces affect the way in which they move. These forces can either be internal – ie inside the athlete's own body – or external – ie outside influences such as gravity and aerodynamics.

A biomechanist will use their knowledge of these disciplines to work out the various factors that affect individuals when performing certain physical movements or activities, such as how water might affect a swimmer's speed or how gravity and air can impact on a long-jumper's performance. Pushing, pulling, lifting, and moving are the sorts of movements that are examined. A detailed analysis of such factors can also help biomechanists advise sportsmen and women on suitable changes they can make to avoid the risk of injury.

Biomechanists carry out analysis by observing how a person moves in their physical activities. Additionally or alternatively, they will also ask them to participate in a series of special tests so that proper assessment can take place, normally with the help of technological equipment such as computer simulation. They will often record their sessions to examine more thoroughly what the individual is doing and to show them ways in which their movement is either slowing them down or causing injury (for example).

Biomechanists don't work just with athletes and

sportspeople, however. They also work more generally with people to help identify and solve – or at least ameliorate – problems that are causing pain and discomfort, such as physical disabilities or injuries. A growing area of development is in surgery, where biomechanics can help in the design of better artificial joints and tissue replacement, for instance.

THE CONDITIONS

Biomechanists work in a variety of locations, from the running track, tennis court and swimming pool, to a local hospital, a special clinic or independently on a self-employed basis. Some lecture on university courses and will, therefore, spend some of their time within an academic setting. Hours can range from a normal working day if spent in a hospital or clinic to long and demanding schedules if you're travelling with a sports team and, for example, attending international competitions. Recent graduates can earn from £18,000 upwards for their first job.

THE ROUTE

Biomechanics is not a subject that you can specialise in at undergraduate level. While it is offered as part of a general sports science degree, you normally will have to do postgraduate study – at masters and/or PhD level – to concentrate solely on this area. Normally, you will need a good honours degree (minimum 2.1) in either sports science or a related area to be accepted on to a course.

THE UPSIDE

The chance to work and travel internationally with sportsmen and women at the top of their career, helping them to achieve their best and stay fit and well, is a big attraction. Helping individuals to live a more comfortable life by assessing their movement and suggesting small ways in which they can change this to relieve pain can be very satisfying and rewarding.

THE DOWNSIDE

The long and potentially unsociable hours if you do work with sports teams or individuals can be tiring and demanding.

FURTHER INFORMATION

- British Association of Sport & Exercise Sciences **www.bases.org.uk**

Which area?

Health promotion specialist

THE WORK

Healthy living is a phrase that's on the tip of everyone's tongue these days, it seems. From Jamie Oliver's school dinners campaign to supermarkets offering vouchers for school sporting equipment, the nation is waking up to the importance of caring for our bodies. The government and the National Health Service are also trying to get us to take control over our own physical and mental well-being but sometimes people need help in knowing how to improve their lives, and this is where health promotions specialists (aka health education specialists or officers) come in.

Normally working in community settings such as schools, hospitals and workplaces, health promotion specialists try to inform people how important it is to take good care of their bodies and minds. This means talking and distributing information about such key

areas as healthy diets and regular exercise, to reduce the risk of obesity and diseases related to it, and the risks of smoking, drinking and unprotected sex.

To get the message out, health promotion specialists also contribute towards marketing campaigns (for example, to flag up the importance of childhood immunisations), producing leaflets, posters and flyers to distribute in health centres, hospitals, libraries and other places easily accessed by the general public. They may even appear on television and radio to raise awareness of their latest campaign. They also work with other key health professionals to implement strategies to improve public health at local, regional and even national levels. Research plays an important role in this as they need to know first the sorts of problems that are emerging in their community and how much the population knows about them.

Working with people obviously is a major part of this job, whether it's running workshops for the local community or meeting with health service managers to discuss future ideas and projects. Liaising with doctors, nurses and other healthcare providers is an essential responsibility.

THE CONDITIONS

Most job vacancies arise with NHS and Primary Care Trusts, although some positions exist in local authorities and relevant charities. However, this is still not a huge field so you'll need to be flexible about location – you may have to move around to find suitable jobs.

Working hours tend to be standard, although you will sometimes need to work at weekends or in the evenings, for example when launching local health initiatives or attending community events. While you will be based in an office, you should be happy to be out and about most of your working day, visiting different people and organisations within your local community.

The salary you can hope to earn is standard with other NHS occupations and ranges from £20,000 to £26,000 per year. This can rise to nearly £40,000 for those with a good deal of experience.

THE ROUTE

Health promotion specialists working in the NHS normally have a degree in biological, social or behavioural sciences. Alternatively, they might have studied for a masters degree in a related area. Experience can count for a lot in this field too, with nursing, social work, medicine, and teaching in a similar area all welcomed. Paid or voluntary work experience also shows that you understand what the work involves and are committed to the area as a whole. If you don't already offer a relevant

postgraduate qualification when you apply for a job, you would normally be expected to study for one within a year or so of taking up a post.

THE UPSIDE

Seeing the benefits of a healthy eating campaign on the health of a local community and the individuals you advise.

THE DOWNSIDE

The paucity of jobs means a steady career route is currently something of an unknown.

FURTHER INFORMATION

- NHS Careers
  www.nhscareers.nhs.uk

Which area?

Occupational therapist

THE WORK

Occupational health is a term bandied about in offices a lot but not many people know exactly what it means. Put simply, occupational therapists try to enable their clients to return to a life of normality after physical or emotional problems, encouraging them to be independent and confident. This could be by looking at ways in which a severely depressed individual could reintegrate themselves into society again or coming up with plans so that an employer can adapt their office space to accommodate a member of staff who is permanently disabled.

Because the problems they deal with can be quite complex, occupational therapists mainly work with clients on an individual basis to ensure that what they recommend is the best strategy. After the initial assessment, occupational therapists will continue monitoring progress, making any changes as appropriate and liaising with the client's family, friends and employers to ensure everyone's needs are being met as closely as possible. Sometimes these goals can be achieved after a few meetings, but more often you will be involved for several months and occasionally longer.

With degenerative diseases such as multiple sclerosis, you will find that the client's problems will change over time. It can be difficult for them to stay positive in light of what is happening to them but a key responsibility of an occupational therapist will be to help motivate them despite this, and gently encourage them to be as active as they can for as long as they can.

THE CONDITIONS

Occupational therapists have a pretty normal working week – around 9am–5pm, Monday to Friday, although part-time work is also possible. They are based in a variety of places, from hospitals, health clinics and GP surgeries to homes, workplaces and schools. Therefore, an ability and willingness to travel, certainly within the local area, is essential.

The starting salary ranges from £20,000 to £26,000 per year, with more experienced practitioners earning over £38,300. With extra experience comes extra opportunities. You could choose to specialise in such areas as paediatrics, mental health, cardiac care, stroke rehabilitation or burns and plastic surgery. Occupational therapists tend to work in multi-disciplinary teams, alongside other health professionals, including nurses, doctors, social workers and physiotherapists.

Currently, the future looks very bright for occupational therapists. NHS Careers states that demand is high for practitioners in this area and it is likely to keep on growing, so you shouldn't encounter any problems getting a job after qualifying.

THE ROUTE

Most people who go into this area do so after undertaking a three-year BSc in occupational health. However, if you'd rather study something else to keep your options open, a two-year accelerated course is offered to graduates from other disciplines. This will lead to a recognised qualification and registration to work either in the NHS or with social services.

THE UPSIDE

Helping someone who has been physically and/or emotionally hurt by accident or illness lead a more fulfilling life.

THE DOWNSIDE

The relatively low pay, although occupational therapists can, with experience, move into managerial posts within the NHS, for example, which would command a higher salary.

FURTHER INFORMATION

- NHS Careers
  www.nhscareers.nhs.uk
- British Association/College of Occupational Therapists
  www.cot.co.uk

Which area?

Physiotherapist

THE WORK

A physiotherapist is someone trained to help people of all ages prevent or recover from all sorts of physical complaints. This could range from helping a person who has undergone extensive surgery become mobile again, to training women how to strengthen their core muscles after having a baby. They will look at such issues as a client's lifestyle, state of mind, physical surroundings and general health, to work out an appropriate prevention or treatment plan, before working closely alongside their clients to meet and maintain these goals successfully.

Much of the remedial work done with patients involves:
- manual therapy, eg helping patients with chest problems after surgery breathe more comfortably and efficiently

- therapeutic exercises, in which the physiotherapist designs certain stretches or movements that will help a patient regain strength or mobility
- electro-physical methods of treatment, such as pain-management systems like TENS machines and ultrasound.

The work is very hands-on and a practical approach is essential. However, you'll also need to be sensitive to the various factors that might influence a person's health and well-being (eg social, emotional and cultural factors). Therefore, you will need a compassionate and empathetic nature, patience to deal with issues that might take a long time to resolve, and the ability to work well in a team alongside other health professionals.

THE CONDITIONS

Physiotherapists are important members of health teams and, as such, can be found working in virtually all hospital departments with doctors and nurses. Most hospitals also have special physiotherapy gyms, where patients can undergo therapeutic exercises and hydrotherapy as part of their rehabilitation. Outpatients are also treated in these areas, receiving ultrasound therapy and advice on posture and movement.

However, it is also becoming increasingly common for individuals to seek out a private physiotherapist to avoid long waiting lists, so employment in private clinics is growing, with physiotherapists working either as part of a team or on their own. Additionally, physiotherapists work in various places in which an accident or injury can occur, from workplaces to leisure centres and educational establishments.

The pay is comparable with other healthcare professionals, with newly qualified practitioners earning anything from £20,000 to £26,000 with the NHS, rising to over £38,000 for more senior posts. An average working week is around 37 hours, Monday to Friday, but if you choose to work in private practice you may find your hours more attuned to your clients' timetables than your own preferences.

With experience, physiotherapists can move on from more general practice to specialise in such areas as care of the elderly, looking after individuals with learning disabilities, or supporting terminally ill patients. Teaching and research are also popular areas. Some people move out of physiotherapy and into health service management.

THE ROUTE

In order to qualify as a physiotherapist, you will need to study for a three- or four-year BSc degree in the subject. Following successful completion of this, you are eligible for registration, which every physiotherapist must attain before being accepted to work in the NHS. Your clinical experience will commence (or continue) after graduation and, at a later date, you will be able to specialise in the area that most appeals to you.

THE UPSIDE

Helping people to live more active and pain-free lives than they might otherwise without your help, and enabling them to learn how to walk again or perform other activities.

THE DOWNSIDE

The work might be physically demanding and tiring at times.

FURTHER INFORMATION

- NHS Careers
  www.nhscareers.nhs.uk
- The Chartered Society of Physiotherapy
  www.csp.org.uk

Which area?

Podiatrist

THE WORK

Here's a surprising fact for you. According to NHS Careers, around 75 to 80% of adults will, at some time in their life, have a problem with their feet, ankles or lower limbs. This means business for podiatrists (aka chiropodists), who specialise in assessing, diagnosing and treating problems in these areas.

This might sound more serious than it is, but don't worry! Problems can range from chronic arthritis, in which a podiatrist will play a palliative role, helping to relieve and manage pain, to a pesky ingrown toenail, which might require a little local anaesthetic while the podiatrist alleviates or removes it. Sometimes, podiatrists just help a person maintain healthy feet, cutting toenails and removing hard skin when their client can't reach these areas. Although many clients are elderly, problems can affect anyone, from a toddler or baby requiring an artificial limb to allay pain or injury, to a person who has become a victim of fashion through wearing impractical heels!

Biomechanics (see page 16) plays a role in podiatry, with practitioners using its principles to work out why a person is having problem with their feet or lower legs. Podiatrists can, therefore, deal with sports injuries and there is great demand for qualified practitioners in this area to help with recovering athletes' rehabilitation.

THE CONDITIONS

According to the Society of Chiropodists and Podiatrists, those graduating with a podiatry degree stand an excellent chance of finding a job within six months of leaving university – around 83% of graduates achive this. They'll work in a variety of settings, from NHS clinics and hospitals, GP surgeries and patient's homes, to private centres, and on a freelance basis. Some podiatrists work in leisure centres and in shops specialising in footwear. More specialised fields include research, academia and the quite new field of forensic podiatry. Podiatrists normally start off undertaking more general work for a while before moving on to specialise in one of the many areas where their services are in demand. However, it is possible to remain more general if this would suit your interests more.

The nature of the work lends itself well to flexible hours, such as part time and flexitime, although you might have to work outside the normal 9am-5pm existence, particularly if you are self-employed, to fit in with your clients' busy schedules. Salaries vary, but are typically around £19,500 for a recently qualified podiatrist with the NHS, rising to £90,000 for consultants.

THE ROUTE

To qualify as a podiatrist you will need to undertake a three- or four-year full-time (or four-and-a-half-year part-time) degree course at an approved university. Around half of the course is theoretical, with the other half involving clinical experience. On graduating, you will normally start off in general practice before moving on to a specialism such as diabetes, paediatrics, biomechanics, rheumatology and dermatology, if you so choose.

THE UPSIDE

The excellent job prospects, the range of people you deal with, and the flexibility this area offers are all attractive reasons to enter this profession.

THE DOWNSIDE

If you want a job with very regular hours this might not be for you, especially if you want to run your own practice. Also, some people hate the idea of working with feet!

FURTHER INFORMATION

- The Society of Chiropodists and Podiatrists
  www.feetforlife.org/careers
- NHS Careers
  www.nhscareers.nhs.uk

Which area?

Prosthetist/Orthotist

THE WORK

Apart from both having names which are difficult words to pronounce, prosthetists and orthotists have other similarities. They work with similar clients, in similar settings, and using similar skills and knowledge. However, there is one important distinction between the two.

A prosthetist is responsible for designing and fitting artificial limbs (called 'prostheses') for people who have lost their own limbs through illness or injury, or were born without the limbs in place. An orthotist, on the other hand, specialises in designing and fitting support items such as braces, collars and splints, which are normally used to help people during the recovery period after injuries and surgery. These 'orthoses' will either be needed on a temporary or permanent basis and will help the client move in a better and less painful way.

Prosthetists and orthotists work with a variety of people with different problems, such as arthritis, cerebral palsy, diabetes and strokes. In order to provide the best possible care, they will need to make a full and careful assessment of the client and their problem, including relevant measurements, before fitting a limb or an orthosis. To do this accurately, a sound knowledge of physiology, anatomy, biomechanics and technology is essential, and normally gained at degree level or higher.

Once the measurements have been taken, the prosthetist/orthotist will liaise with a technician to explain their designs and ideas before he or she begins to make them. Once the limb or orthosis is ready, a fitting will take place, and the prosthetist/orthotist will conduct regular check-ups to ensure that everything is going well and that the client is managing. Sometimes adjustments or minor repairs will need to be made.

As well as working with patients, prosthetists and orthotists also liaise with physiotherapists and occupational therapists to give the client suitable exercise regimes and to adapt to life with their new prosthesis or orthosis.

THE CONDITIONS

Professionals working in these fields are normally based in hospitals or in special physical rehabilitation centres. A standard working week will be around 37 to 40 hours long, from Monday to Friday. Many can and do work part time. Typical starting salaries are £20,000–£25,000 per year, rising to £40,000 for those with considerable experience.

Graduates looking for a career in this area will not be disappointed. According to the British Association of Prosthetists and Orthotists, there is a worldwide shortage in these areas so prospects are fantastic. Jobs for newly qualified orthotists and prosthetists are normally found in the public sector – in the NHS – or in the private sector – in manufacturing companies. International work is also possible, especially with charities that help people injured in wars and other crises. At higher levels, prothetists and orthotists can take on teaching roles or managerial positions, and there will also be opportunities to work in research and development.

THE ROUTE

The normal route to a career in this area is to complete a four-year degree course that has been approved by the Health Professionals Council (HPC). This will enable you to be eligible for registration, an essential requirement to practise in this field. The degree will combine a mixture of academic/theoretic learning (encompassing such areas as life sciences, biomechanics, engineering and material sciences and prosthetic and orthotic sciences, as well as mathematics and IT) and practical hands-on experience at local hospitals.

THE UPSIDE

The variety: these jobs are so fascinating because they combine both technical and analytical skills with the regular client contact.

THE DOWNSIDE

The salaries aren't huge but they're not bad either. There aren't many prosthetics/orthotics courses out there so competition to get on one could be fierce.

FURTHER INFORMATION

- NHS Careers
  www.nhscareers.nhs.uk
- British Association of Prosthetists and Orthotists
  www.bapo.com

Which area?

Sports and exercise psychologist

THE WORK

Imagine being faced with a stadium full of people and feeling the pressure to become the fastest sprinter in the world. How would you cope under that pressure? Would you use it to your advantage – using that adrenaline to make you run faster? Or would nerves get the better of you, possibly making you stumble or leave the block before the gun has been fired?

The mind can have a profound effect on the body. Sports and exercise psychologists study this relationship and apply it in a practical way to help sportspeople perform to the best of their ability. They help sportspeople prepare psychologically for competition in the following ways:

- teaching relaxation techniques so that energy is not wasted in an unhelpful way

- practising visualisation exercises – if you see yourself winning a race, your confidence levels should rise
- increasing levels of confidence – if you don't think you can score a winning goal, you probably won't
- instilling a positive attitude that won't flag when the going gets tough.

Sports and exercise psychologists can also share their insights and knowledge with coaches so they can help to motivate, not discourage, their athletes.

A growing field is looking at how the mind–body relationship works the other way around. It is generally accepted these days that exercise releases feel-good endorphins so physical activity can be incredibly beneficial in helping people to overcome mental illnesses such as depression.

Sports psychologists work with a wide range of people too – from amateurs to professionals, individuals to teams, coaches to referees, and ordinary people who aren't very sports focused but for whom activity would prove beneficial, including both adults and children.

THE CONDITIONS

Sports and exercise psychologists may work from an office or clinic but they are just as likely to be found travelling locally, nationally and internationally, wherever the need for their services is felt, often in sporting venues. Some find employment with a national sport governing body, while others lecture in universities. Most sports psychologists do a combination of consultancy and teaching because, while their services are in increasing demand, there still aren't enough vacancies for the number of applicants. Therefore, you'll probably find yourself working in a bizarre variety of settings, from a comfortable office or clinic to a freezing, wet rugby pitch!

Your earning capability will depend on how experienced you are and who your clients are. A recently qualified psychologist in this field normally earns from £20,000 upwards, while a team psychologist could expect £30,000 and above, together with a car and any expenses related to travelling. Psychologists working in academia earn from £21,000 to £32,000 or more.

THE ROUTE

It takes quite a while to qualify as a sports psychologist. Normally you will need to have completed either an undergraduate degree in psychology or a postgraduate conversion course, both of which should allow you to be eligible for the Graduate Basis for Registration (GBR). After this, you will need to undertake a further three years of postgraduate training, with supervision and clinical placements.

THE UPSIDE

Working with a wide variety of people in a range of settings, helping them to achieve their best mentally and/or physically.

THE DOWNSIDE

The training can be quite demanding, mentally and financially, especially when there are fewer jobs than there are graduates.

FURTHER INFORMATION

- British Association of Sport & Exercise Sciences
  www.bases.org.uk
- British Psychological Society
  www.bps.org.uk

Which area?

Sports and exercise scientist

THE WORK

It might seem strange to combine science with sports but this is exactly what this career and study area does. So how are the two linked?

Sports and exercise scientists help both athletes and members of the general public improve their abilities and overall health through physical activity. They do this by applying principles from such diverse disciplines as physiology and psychology to influence positively the way in which a person can move or think or behave, helping them to recover from injuries, preventing illnesses and achieving the best of their ability no matter what their standard of fitness.

As such, working with people plays a major role in this career. You could be dealing with a wide variety of individuals, from other sports experts such as coaches and therapists, to doctors and other health professionals, individual athletes and teams. Your remit might be quite broad too – for example, liaising with Primary Care Trusts to come up with rehabilitative exercise programmes. There may also be work on research projects and invitations from sports goods companies to help design sports equipment.

THE CONDITIONS

Sports, health and wellbeing are high on the social and political agendas at the moment so, in theory, opportunities in this area should be good. However, while it can't be denied that this field is on the up, there are still not many vacancies around and competition for the few that are there is fierce. These can normally be found in such places as universities, health services, and private and public sporting organisations; or perhaps you'd rather work on a freelance basis, running your own business and working with athletes and teams. A degree and experience in this area could also help you become involved in related fields such as sports development and performance testing.

Working hours are normal, at around 38 per week. However, you might find some of these falling at weekends and evenings, to work around your clients' commitments, so antisocial hours are fairly common. Most sports scientists work from consultation rooms but some outdoor work is also possible, depending on the work you are undertaking with your clients.

An average salary in this area is about £20,000 to £40,000 per year, depending on experience, your employer and how busy you are. If you are lucky enough to get work with clients who are at the top of their field, you might take home £60,000 per year or more. Suffice it to say, people who do this job do it more for a love of their chosen area than the lure of wealth.

THE ROUTE

Most people who work in this field come into it with a sports science degree, although it is also acceptable to have a qualification in a related field and then do a postgraduate course. Since competition is tough in this area, it is a good idea to get some experience in sports coaching or working perhaps as a fitness instructor, both of which could provide a valuable foot in the door.

THE UPSIDE

Imagine seeing an athlete win a race because of your advice!

THE DOWNSIDE

The opportunities are still few and far between and the ones that do exist don't command a mind-boggling pay packet.

FURTHER INFORMATION

- British Association of Sports and Exercise Sciences (BASES)
  www.bases.org.uk
- Skills Active
  www.skillsactive.com

Which area?

Sports coach

THE WORK

Sports coaches have been represented in a variety of ways on television and films – not normally in a very complimentary light! Often shown as being loud, aggressive, dictatorial and cruel, this portrayal is far from the truth. Their main job is to help individuals and teams of various standards, from the local under-tens football team to an Olympic 100-metre sprinter, to perform to the best of their ability.

Individuals all respond differently to motivation, so a sports coach must be able to decide what method would best suit their client(s), using their extensive knowledge to advise on how to win a game or improve a time. Most of this takes place in training sessions before major events but a coach will be there on the day to offer support. Understanding how people think and interact with one another is a very important part of

the job, as is identifying when a particular approach is not bringing about the desired results.

To make sure they are providing the very best for their athletes, coaches also seek assistance from outside their own area of expertise. For example, they may liaise with nutritionists to come up with suitable diets, or with physiotherapists to discuss training options after injury. And, with money being increasingly important in the world of sport, coaches may find themselves trying to negotiate sponsorship details with local, national or even international companies to help fund the training and travelling their sportsmen and women undertake.

THE CONDITIONS

Sporting events take place at all times of the day and night, at weekends and during public holidays, so say goodbye to a 'normal' working week if you want to specialise in this area! That said, some coaches are able to work part time, while others just work seasonally – eg in the summer at special sports camps for children and teenagers.

You won't be sitting in a comfortable office either. Your working locations may vary between schools and universities to local or national sports centres – wherever your athletes are training. This could be a swimming pool, a running track, a football pitch or in a sweaty gym. While you won't be competing yourself, you will still need to have a good standard of physical health and strength in order to cope with long training times and demonstrating techniques to sportspeople. Travel is also possible – even probable – in this job.

Unfortunately the pay isn't much to write home about. It is estimated that newly-qualified coaches might earn anywhere between £10,000 and £14,000 working for local authorities, while more experienced individuals can earn over £30,000 if employed by a national governing body. A few of the lucky ones, normally those coaching athletes competing at international level, will earn more than £100,000 per year. If you choose to work on a self-employed basis, the sort of hourly rate you could expect is from £15 to £60. Many coaches offer their services voluntarily too.

THE ROUTE

Some sports coaches don't have a degree but it is becoming common for people interested in a career in this area to study for one in a related area. However, this alone will not make you eligible to become a coach; you will need to obtain the appropriate coaching qualification by your chosen sport's national governing body. Some degrees incorporate coaching qualifications into them, so it's worth trying to find this out when applying.

Practice is as important as theory though so you will need to show a commitment to sports coaching by taking part in it. Voluntary opportunities, such as coaching a children's football team, are a good place to start.

THE UPSIDE

If you love sport and working with people, what better combination could you hope for?

THE DOWNSIDE

The salary – if you're not working with the big shots you might need another job to pay the bills.

FURTHER INFORMATION

- SkillsActive
  www.skillsactive.com/careers
- Sports Coach UK
  www.sportscoachuk.org

Which area?

Sports development officer (SDO)

THE WORK

As concern over levels of obesity in the UK grows, health professionals want to ensure that both adults and children have access to sports and other physical activities in their area to help keep them healthy. This is where a sports development officer comes in. He or she will work alongside local councils, schools, clubs and other organisations, such as the police and national governing bodies, to ensure that opportunities are available and that everyone knows about them.

A large part of their job will be identifying the different sectors of society that might need extra help and support in getting involved, including people from disadvantaged backgrounds, individuals with physical or emotional disabilities, the elderly and the very young. This will normally mean coming up with suitable ways to reach out to them, such as liaising with the police, social workers, health professionals, teachers and local charities so their message gets out.

Additionally, SDOs recruit and train volunteers to help out on schemes, such as after-school clubs and holiday activities, and try to source funding to enable these groups to run. Much of the work tends to be administrative rather than sporty in nature, as the latter is left to the volunteers and any coaches who come on board. Therefore, SDOs can often be found writing reports, maintaining databases, assessing projects, marketing opportunities and finding funding. A suit would probably be worn more often than a tracksuit!

THE CONDITIONS

Working hours depend on who your employer is. If you land a job with a local authority, it's standard to work a 36-hour week, although you may have to attend meetings or events outside of these. The good news is that extra work will probably be paid or time in lieu given. You will normally be office-based though you will normally also have meetings out and about with people who are either supporting or using your schemes and initiatives, often in schools and other clubs. Be ready to work in all sorts of weathers and conditions too, especially if you are attending a rainy Bank Holiday footie match!

As with other professionals in the sporting arena, the money isn't much to write home about. A typical starting salary with a local authority can be around £16,700 per year, rising to £24,000 with a few more years' experience. More senior roles can command salaries in excess of £40,000.

The better news is that the demand for SDOs will be increasing with the London Olympics in 2012. Vacancies will spring up throughout the UK, not just in the capital, and will typically be found in local authorities seeking to put sport higher on their agenda.

THE ROUTE

There is no set degree requirement to get into this area but admittedly employers might find you a more attractive candidate if you can offer a degree in a related subject such as sports science or management. You won't need to go on to further postgraduate study (unless you want to, of course!) but work experience is vital to show commitment and knowledge of what's entailed. Voluntary work is often a great way in, so check out local opportunities at home and at university to help with coaching or teaching sports.

THE UPSIDE

Using your knowledge of and commitment to sport to help often disadvantaged people become healthier and happier in life.

THE DOWNSIDE

Don't expect to be driving a Ferrari on this salary (but with your interest in health promotion, you'll be cycling anyway, right?)

FURTHER INFORMATION

- Sports Leaders UK
  www.sportsleaders.org
- The Institute of Sport and Recreation Management (ISRM)
  www.isrm.co.uk

www.ucas.com

helping students into higher education

The career for you?

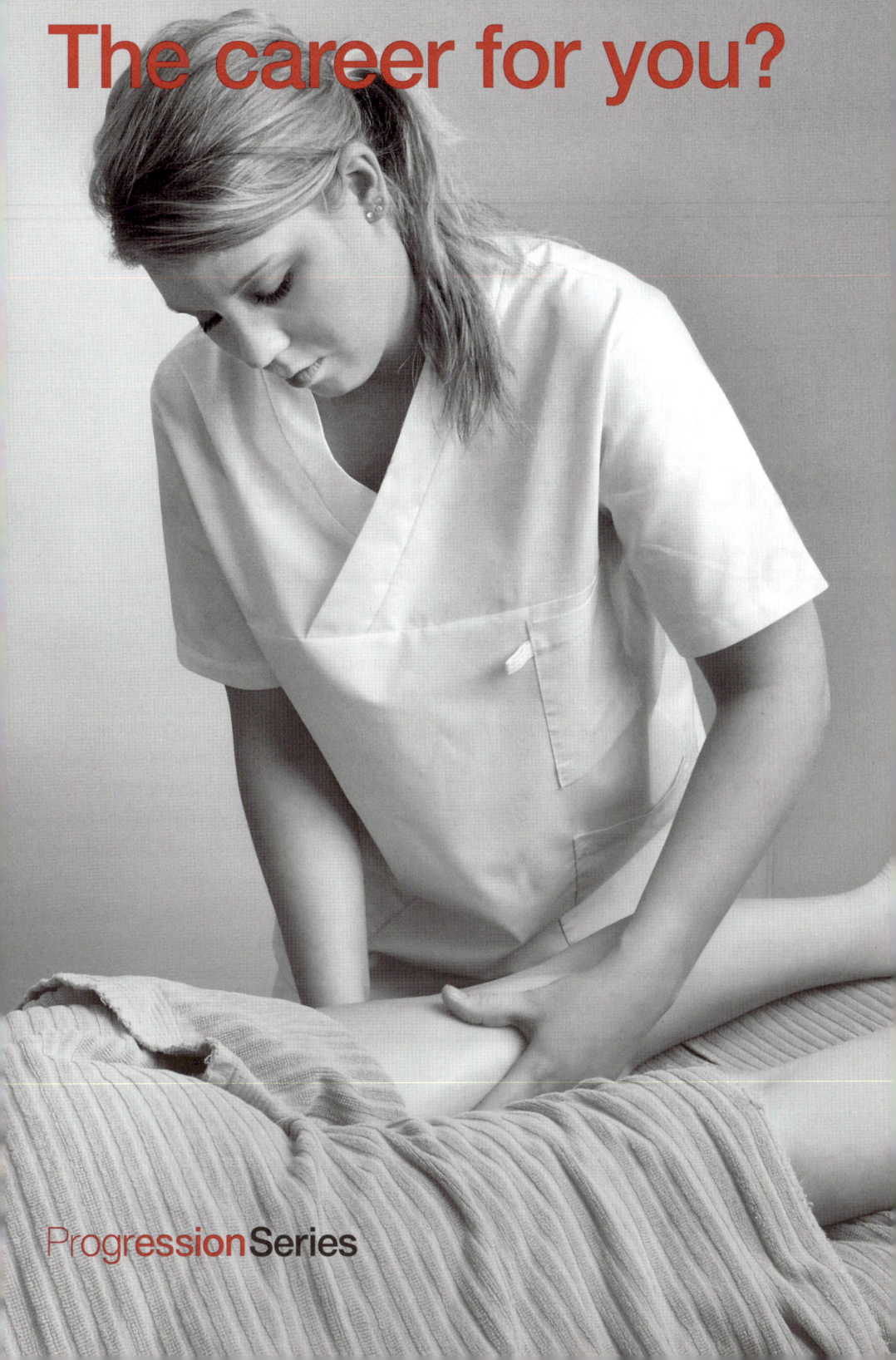

Is sports science and physiotherapy for you?

Being successful – in whatever specialism – calls for more than an in-depth understanding of the relevant discipline; it also requires certain skills and personal qualities or attributes.

To help you decide if a career in a sports science-related area is for you, we suggest you consider the following questions:

- What do you want from your future work?
- What does the course typically involve?
- Which skills do professionals in sports science-related areas and physiotherapy typically need?

WHAT DO YOU WANT FROM YOUR FUTURE CAREER?

You may not have an instant answer for this now, but your current studies, work experience to date and even your hobbies can help give you clues about the kind of work you enjoy, and the skills you have already started to develop. Start with a blank sheet of paper and note down your answers to the questions we've asked below to help get you thinking. Be as brutally honest with yourself as you can. Don't write what you think will impress your teachers or parents; write what really matters to you and you'll start to see a pattern emerge.

ANSWER THESE QUESTIONS TO HELP YOU CHOOSE YOUR CAREER

- When you think of your future, in what kind of environment do you see yourself working: office, outdoor, 9am-5pm, high-pressure, regular routine?
- What are your favourite hobbies outside school?
- What is it about them you enjoy? Working with people, working out how things work?
- What are your favourite subjects at school?
- What is it about them that you enjoy most? Being able to create something, debating, problem solving, practical hands-on work?
- What do you dislike about the other subjects you're studying? (Writing 'the teacher' doesn't count!)
- Which aspects of your work experience have you most enjoyed?

WHICH SKILLS WILL YOU TYPICALLY NEED?

Without doubt, admissions tutors in sports science look for applicants who love sport and who want to learn about how it can improve people's lives. Therefore, clear **evidence of a commitment to sports** as a career is essential, which can usually be demonstrated through work experience placements with charitable organisations, for example, and participation in individual and/or team sports. This will also provide proof of your **ability to work well and get on with a wide variety of people**. Teamwork is an essential part of any sports science-related career, whether working with sportspeople or with other professionals supporting them, so you will need to show that you relish opportunities to work as part of a wider initiative. However, an interest in sports and people won't cut it without a **good academic record**. People often believe that they don't need high GCSE and A level grades to get on in sports. However, this is not the case and it is very likely that offers will become even higher in the future with more applicants fighting for places.

This is also true for careers in podiatry and physiotherapy. When people come to you with physical problems, they may also want to talk more generally about their lives and how any disabilities or illnesses they may have impact on that. Therefore, a **sympathetic nature and good listening skills** are vital. This is equally applicable for sports and exercise psychologists, who spend much of their time listening and relating to their clients in order to work out how best to help them through their issues. Therefore (as is also the case with all other sports science-related areas), an **analytical approach** is indispensable – you will need some sort of distance from the problems and puzzles you face to come up with workable solutions.

Finally, you must not forget that sports science, physiotherapy, podiatry and psychology are very much **science-based subjects**, so an interest in the relevant fields is essential. It is not uncommon for universities offering these subjects to ask for at least one A level in a science subject such as biology, chemistry or physics. Sciences also demand a very particular approach to their study, and the following 'hard' skills will be vital:

- excellent problem-solving
- a logical approach to looking at issues
- an analytical outlook to cope with statistical information
- a methodical approach to your work
- computer literacy.

ALTERNATIVE CAREERS

While many graduates progress into a sports-related field after university, some will decide to change direction. A sports science degree will develop your analytical thinking abilities and problem-solving skills, which are in demand in many different professions, including management, sales, marketing and other related fields within the leisure industry and beyond. Your people skills and teamworking ability will make you an attractive candidate for a career in personnel and human resources, should that area appeal to you. Sports might be the 'be all' for you at the moment but if you change your mind during your degree they need not be the 'end all'.

Graduate destinations

Each year, comprehensive statistics are collected on what graduates are doing six months after they complete their course. The survey is co-ordinated by the Higher Education Statistics Agency (HESA) and provides information about how many graduates move into employment (and what type of career) or further study and how many are believed to be unemployed.

The full results across all subject areas are published by the Higher Education Careers Service Unit (HECSU) and the Association of Graduate Careers Advisory Services (AGCAS) in *What Do Graduates Do?,* which is available from www.ucasbooks.com.

	Sports Science and Physiotherapy
In UK employment	64.8%
In overseas employment	2.0%
Working and studying	8.1%
Studying in the UK for a higher degree	5.2%
Studying in the UK for a teaching qualification	5.1%
Undertaking other further study or training in the UK	3.2%
Studying overseas	0.2%
Not available for employment, study or training	4.4%
Assumed to be unemployed	4.1%
Other	3.0%

Occupation	Percentage
Marketing, Sales and Advertising Professionals	3.0%
Commercial, Industrial and Public Sector Managers	6.9%
Scientific Research, Analysis & Development Professionals	1.2%
Engineering Professionals	0.3%
Health Professionals and Associate Professionals	23.4%
Education Professionals	8.8%
Business and Financial Professionals and Associate Professionals	4.1%
Information Technology Professionals	0.3%
Art, Design, Culture and Sports Professionals	14.6%
Legal Professionals	0.1%
Social & Welfare Professionals	2.4%
Other Professionals, Associate Professional and Technical Occupations	1.8%
Numerical Clerks and Cashiers	1.4%
Other Clerical and Secretarial Occupations	7.2%
Retail, Catering, Waiting and Bar Staff	8.5%
Other Occupations	15.9%
Unknown Occupations	0.1%

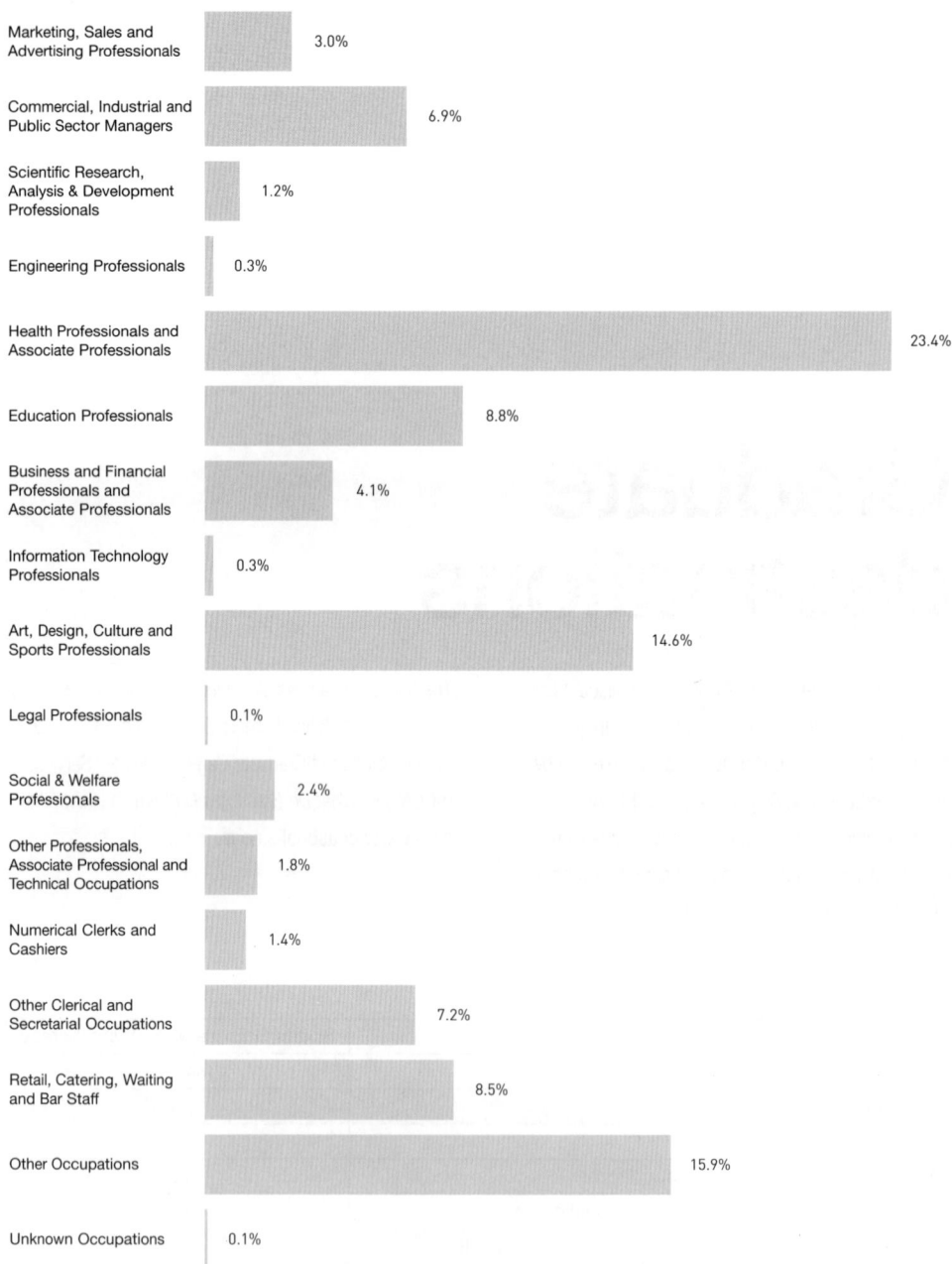

Reproduced with the kind permission of HECSU/AGCAS, *What Do Graduates Do? 2009.*
Data from the HESA Destinations of Leavers of Higher Education Survey 06/07

Case studies

**JUST WHAT DOES A CAREER IN SPORTS
SCIENCE AND RELATED FIELDS OFFER YOU?**

The following profiles show the wealth of exciting
opportunities that are yours for the taking.

Junior physiotherapist

Northampton General Hospital NHS Trust

JENNIFER RILEY

Route into physiotherapy:
A levels – biology, history, geography; AS level chemistry, general studies; BSc physiotherapy, Coventry University
and the University of Leicester (2008)

WHY PHYSIOTHERAPY?

I have been interested in working in a medical
profession from a young age and I also had a huge
interest in teaching. Physiotherapy can combine both
these areas: in my role I work with patients to help with
their rehabilitation and I also teach physiotherapy
students. It is a very diverse career with many differing
prospects, and the career progression and development
opportunities attracted me.

HOW DID YOU GET WHERE YOU ARE TODAY?

I received an unconditional offer from the University of
Leicester. The course was very intense and mixed both
formal and practical teaching and lectures with practical
placements based in a variety of mainly NHS settings.

After qualifying in 2008, I took a temporary contract at
Loughborough General Hospital, working in their
musculoskeletal outpatient department for about two
months. During this time I applied for full-time NHS
posts. I then returned to my home town and began
work in a private clinic before being offered a junior
rotational post at Northampton General Hospital, where I
have been working to date in orthopaedics.

WHAT DOES YOUR JOB INVOLVE?

On a daily basis I work with senior physiotherapists and technical instructors within the hospital's orthopaedic in-patient department. I help with patients' rehabilitation when they are recovering from joint replacements and other orthopaedic surgeries, in both gym and ward sessions. This includes gait re-education, exercises and mobility aid assessments. I am responsible for safely progressing patients with their treatments so they can be discharged from hospital. I also refer patients for further treatment if required.

Being employed in a hospital means working with a wide variety of professionals from different disciplines. Within the physiotherapy department these include senior and junior physiotherapists, technical instructors and physiotherapy assistants. Other professionals I interact with include doctors, nurses, occupational therapists, community physiotherapists, discharge co-ordinators, speech and language therapists, and many more. As I rotate every four months, I will come into contact with varying specialities of other professionals too.

WHAT HAS BEEN YOUR BIGGEST CHALLENGE?

This came when I first took the position at Northampton General. I'd had no previous undergraduate experience within an orthopaedic setting and I was assigned a 28-bed trauma ward to run with the aid of a single technical instructor! It was an excellent learning experience and although initially it felt like being 'thrown in at the deep end' I have since moved onto the elective surgery ward and can see that it was a great learning curve. I did receive support from my seniors but, on a day-to-day basis, it was my responsibility to assess, treat and discharge patients with broken hips safely.

AND THE BEST BITS?

I enjoy my job because it allows to me to spend all day with a wide variety of people, both fellow medical professionals and patients. It gives me huge satisfaction to see the achievements patients make – for instance, a patient who, after not being able to get out of bed unassisted, progresses with our physio team's treatment to walking independently with walking sticks and returning to their own home.

JENNIFER'S TOP TIPS

Get as much pre-application experience as you can. Universities want to see that you're truly interested in this profession so write to hospitals, private practices, sports teams and care centres to gain all the voluntary or paid experience that you can. This will also help you decide if physiotherapy is the career for you.

Senior lecturer, sport and exercise psychology

University of Portsmouth

JENNY PAGE

Route into physiotherapy:

A levels – human biology, psychology, physical education (2000); BSc sport and exercise science, University of Chichester (2003); MSc sport and exercise psychology, University of Chichester (2004); PhD sport psychology, University of Liverpool (2009)

WHY SPORTS PSYCHOLOGY?

I really enjoyed the sports psychology part of my sports science degree: it allowed me to think about factors that I had not previously considered to be very important in performing well, such as being confident, motivated and focused when performing. I then wanted to use my knowledge to help sports performers so I trained to become a sports psychologist.

HOW DID YOU GET TO WHERE YOU ARE TODAY?

As well as the sport psychology modules offered at my university, I also studied at a university in Canada for one semester and this allowed me to take a diverse range of sports psychology modules. I was also lucky enough to be offered some teaching hours for first-year students when I was completing my MSc. During this time, I applied for the supervised experience process through BASES (the British Association of Sport and Exercise Science), which trains sports psychologists. When I had completed my MSc, I applied for and was successful in getting a graduate teaching assistant position at the University of Chester. After the three-year contract had finished I applied for a lecturer position at the University of Portsmouth. I was keen to secure a lecturing job because it would enable me to continue lecturing, researching and doing applied work as a sports psychologist.

WHAT DOES YOUR JOB INVOLVE?

My responsibilities include teaching undergraduate and postgraduate students, providing pastoral care and producing high-quality research. I am also completing my PhD, so I spend time working on this and carrying out other related research. When opportunities arise, I provide psychology support to athletes.

As a lecturer, I teach students from college right through to MSc level, through lectures, seminars and laboratories and my regular working day is normally from 8.00am until 5.30pm during term time. However, both my research and the work I do with athletes are often completed in the evenings and at weekends. As a sports psychologist I have completed workshops with a

Rugby League Academy, Hampshire Gymnastics and the Independent Schools Football Association for Girls. I have also delivered one-to-one consultancy with a rugby union player, rugby league players, shooters and a football referee, amongst other performers.

WHAT HAS BEEN YOUR BIGGEST CHALLENGE?

The biggest challenge I have is ongoing: juggling teaching, my PhD, other research and my work as a sports psychologist. Luckily my colleagues are very supportive and have allowed me time to collect data and write my thesis, while teaching a manageable workload. My work regularly extends beyond office hours.

WHAT DO YOU ENJOY MOST ABOUT YOUR JOB?

I really enjoy educating the students about various aspects of sports psychology, and making them think about their own sporting achievements and how psychology has helped them or may help them in the future. I have also found it satisfying developing my research profile through designing and conducting research with the specific aim of answering questions that will advance the field of sports psychology.

JENNY'S TOP TIPS

If you want to become a lecturer, once you have your degree and are undertaking an MSc, ask your institution if you can help deliver some of the lectures, seminars or laboratories. If you would like to be a sports psychologist, you will need to obtain a postgraduate qualification in the area.

Self-employed personal trainer

Gloucestershire

PAUL WANFORD

Route into personal training:

A levels: sport science, biology and geography; Degree: BSc sport and exercise sciences, University of Gloucestershire (2000)

WHY SPORTS SCIENCE AND EXERCISE?

My choice of degree was initially fuelled by the fact that I have always enjoyed sport from a young age and also that of my 3 A levels sports science was my best result! I realised that working in the fitness industry could be challenging, rewarding and a great way to really change people's lives.

I soon became aware that to progress in the fitness industry there are two routes: management or personal training (or a combination of the two). The management route takes away the essence of the job (as I found out), hence I have stuck to my passion, which is personal training.

HOW DID YOU GET WHERE YOU ARE TODAY?

I graduated in June 2000 and got a job with a chain of sports clubs as a fitness instructor, moving between various centres and working as fitness manager and duty manager for 3 years. I also gained vocational qualifications in this time and started to work as a personal trainer both for my employer and freelance.

In May 2003, I got a job as duty manager at a leisure club in Gloucester, my then plan being to take the management route. This lasted two weeks before I realised my true passion is personal training. I quit (the one and only time I have done this, which felt very wrong!!), spent £250 on 2000 flyers and 1000 business cards and set up Paul Wanford Personal Training in Cheltenham. This was growing very well and in 2006, I joined forces with two other people and became the Fitness Team. One of the other two people has since parted company and we now have four other trainers working for us.

WHAT DOES YOUR JOB INVOLVE?

I spend my time assessing, motivating, progressing and at times annoying clients on a one-to-one or small group basis from their home, office or my small studio.

I will plan and prepare fitness programmes to meet clients' needs and supervise and encourage them to exceed their goals.

I personally get up at 5 am and my first client is at 6am and the last finishes at about 8.30pm. There are gaps within this and as it is not office-based, I spend a lot of time travelling to and from clients.

I have a very diverse client base in terms of age, ability and background which makes for a very interesting and enjoyable diary of sessions.

WHAT HAS BEEN THE BIGGEST CHALLENGE?

The biggest challenge for me has been building a business from scratch 140 miles away from my family home. There have been many sacrifices made and thousands of flyers handed out. But the buzz from knowing you have done it all yourself in an industry that is helping people look after their health, boost their confidence and ultimately prolong their life is awesome!

WHAT DO YOU LIKE MOST ABOUT YOUR JOB?

- I am making a difference to people
- I get to keep fit on the job
- I am my own boss (ish)
- I have made great friends
- Running with clients past a queue of traffic full of people all off to the office makes it even better
- Being taken on holiday!

PAUL'S TOP TIPS

- Learn your trade with a big gym company - you will get looked after and meet some great people.
- It is a customer-based service, so never be late and remember the customer is always right (sometimes).

Clinical Lead, Musculoskeletal Podiatry

Cwm Taf NHS Trust and Private practice

GAFIN MORGAN

Route into podiatry:

A levels: biology, psychology, science engineering and technology foundation; BSc (Hons) Podiatry, University of Wales - UWIC, 1997

WHY PODIATRY?

I wanted to work in an area of healthcare that was specialised in some way to one area of the body and where I could work with all ages and with various types of problems eg sports, paediatrics, elderly etc. Also, I wanted to work in a healthcare profession that allowed me to keep learning throughout my career and one which I found stimulating. In particular I enjoy working with sports injuries and have found podiatry allows me to do this very successfully. It is a vital aspect of healthcare in sports medicine.

I have been in practice for over ten years now and it has been a mix of natural progression and my own determination which has resulted in my being in my present role. My current role in the NHS has provided me with development of various skills including team work, leadership, and management and of course clinical. I can decide quite freely on the direction of the musculoskeletal podiatry service and seeing good results is very rewarding. Overall I treat slightly more sports people in private practice than with my NHS work, however, the percentage is not a great deal more.

HOW DID YOU GET WHERE YOU ARE TODAY?

Since graduation I have worked in the private and public sector and decided on my area of interest within podiatry quite quickly ie musculoskeletal podiatry and sports injuries. I have worked towards this goal continuously since, gaining experience in this field by learning form my colleagues, attending postgraduate courses and by constantly applying learning in my daily role.

WHAT DOES YOUR JOB INVOLVE?

My work involves treating patients with lower limb musculoskeletal problems and managing a team of specialist podiatrists in the same field. I run specialist clinics which involve biomechanical assessments of patients, requesting diagnostics (eg x-rays, MRI, ultrasound), using various treatment methods eg acupuncture, muscle balance exercises and foot orthoses. I also manage fifty-six clinical sessions per week which is a pretty busy! I work 37.5 hours per week for the NHS and an additional 5 or so hours privately. Working hours are from 8:45am until 5:15pm for the NHS.

I am also responsible for the health and safety of staff and for ensuring their knowledge and skills are up to date. This means that I often need to have a very good overview of a specialist area of podiatry practice. I work alone at clinic and with other healthcare professionals. I work one day a week with a physiotherapist and one day per week with an orthopaedic consultant. These clinics are very interesting and we learn a great deal from each other. I also liaise with other professionals eg radiologists, rheumatologists and not forgetting cleaners without whom we would not be able to work!

WHAT HAS BEEN YOUR BIGGEST CHALLENGE?

I continually encounter various challenges which encourage me to develop my skills and thinking, ranging from leadership challenges to specific clinical challenges. Working out the logistics of my clinical team and how I can achieve waiting list targets would be a good example of my leadership challenges. To complete this task involved a good understanding of the skills of five clinical specialists, availability of clinical rooms, and liaising with other clinical staff.

One of my greatest clinical challenges was treating an Olympic athlete for the first time. The amount of responsibility in treating this particular athlete was significant as his performance was very much dependant on my treatment. The treatment involved a complex biomechanical assessment of the athlete's gait and foot function with the prescription of a functional foot orthotic which is a custom insole that alters foot and limb function. All of this needed to happen within a 48-hour period.

WHAT DO YOU LIKE MOST ABOUT YOUR JOB?

This is difficult to summarise but I think most of all when a patient tells you that they are pain-free and what you have done has changed their life. I also enjoy the possibilities of being able to apply my skills and knowledge to help sportspeople perform better. You can almost share in the successes of their sport, which is a great feeling.

GAFIN'S TOP TIPS

I would recommend visiting a podiatrist in practice and try to get some idea what it may be like to work as a podiatrist. Try and visit various podiatry practices as our scope of practice is surprisingly large. But remember at the same time that your career path and development are entirely of to your own making.

Prosthetist

Opcare Ltd

MOOSE BAXTER

Route into prosthetics:
A levels – Maths, Biology, Chemistry; BSc Prosthetics and Orthotics, Strathclyde (2007)

WHY PROSTHETICS?

I always knew that I wanted to work in a caring profession. I was first attracted to prosthetics and orthotics due to the range of study that it involves. Engineering principles, life sciences, anatomy and the hands-on manufacturing of artificial limbs are all combined, which sounded like something I would enjoy.

HOW DID YOU GET WHERE YOU ARE TODAY?

A man in a pub suggested prosthetics and orthotics! I looked into this, and found the idea very interesting. I had never excelled in any one particular subject more than another, so the opportunity to bring together lots of different aspects really attracted me. I put in my application, got through the course (including a year on clinical placements) and following graduation I got a job as a prosthetist, where I have been given much ongoing support. Each day is a new and interesting challenge with real, visible results, such as enabling patients to walk again following amputation.

WHAT DOES YOUR JOB INVOLVE?

As a prosthetist, I run out-patient hospital clinics for amputees and people with congenital limb deficiencies. My role involves working with the multi-disciplinary team to assess new patients and prescribe suitable artificial limbs or useful components for their existing prostheses. I then take detailed measurements and a plaster of Paris cast of the patient's residual limb and work with technicians to custom make an artificial arm or leg. CAD CAM is playing an increasing role in our daily work, and it's exciting to see the other developments and technologies that are gradually becoming available for use. Once patients are referred to us, we continue to see them for ongoing prosthetic care for as long as they continue to wear an artificial limb.

WHAT HAS BEEN YOUR BIGGEST CHALLENGE?

It can be hard convincing patients that we have their best interests in mind when discussing which type of artificial limb would be most suitable for them. For example, we would be unlikely to give a leg designed for sprinting to an 85-year-old person who hasn't sprinted for 50 years. An inappropriate limb prescription would be unsafe and they'd probably struggle to walk on it. Instead, we'll make a limb that will help them stand and begin to re-learn to walk. Although this can be very challenging, the fact that we work with the patient to achieve the best results is very satisfying.

WHAT DO YOU LIKE MOST ABOUT YOUR JOB?

What I like most about prosthetics is that every day can be a challenge. One day there may be an unusual case that requires input from many members of the clinical team. The next day all the patients attending could be in the department for hours, needing lots done to their artificial limbs and I'm rushing round all day. Other days, newly available components and products may be demonstrated, or I'm fitting one of them for the first time. Some days are less exciting than others, but helping people to walk again is something that I expect to continue to enjoy for a long time!

MOOSE'S TOP TIPS

Look into the course and know what to expect when enrolling. It's hard work, but very rewarding! Speak to prosthetists and orthotists locally about the course and their job. Don't expect to get a job in a specific location immediately after graduation. Although the number of graduate opportunities equates fairly closely to the number of graduates, jobs are spread across the UK.

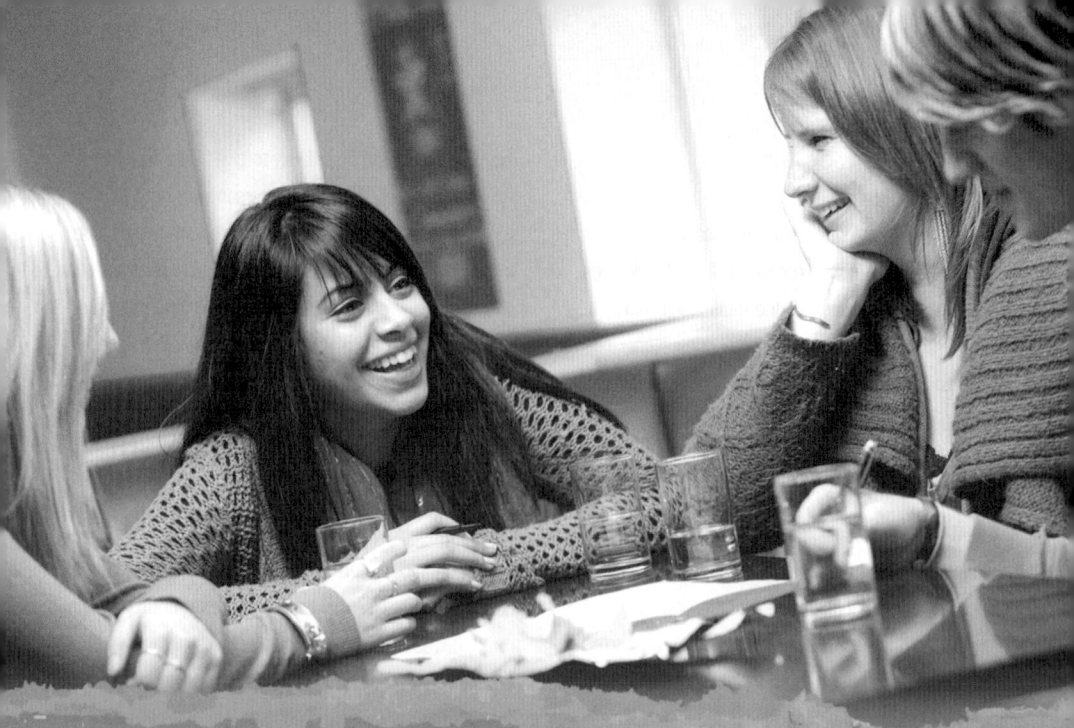

Entry routes

a parent?

get the facts about higher education

Exclusive parents' website

To find out all about higher education and the application process, log on to our new website, exclusively for parents.

Free guide for parents

For a wealth of information about finance, student welfare and selecting the right course and university or college, register online and receive your free copy of the Parent Guide and bi-monthly email bulletins.

Register today at www.ucas.com/parents

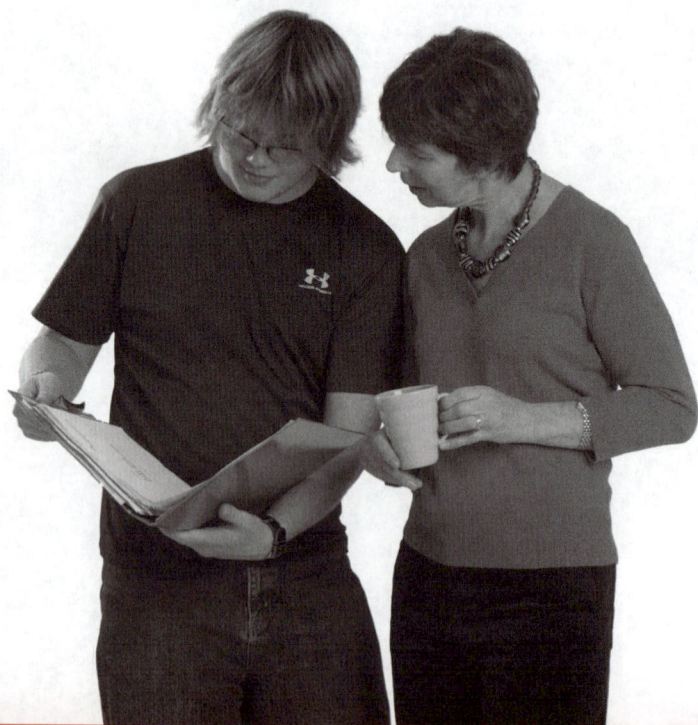

Routes to qualification

Sports science-related subjects are many and varied, making it impossible to cover all the various routes to qualifications here. The **Areas of work** profiles on pages 16–35 give a brief summary of what is required in each of the highlighted professions so take a look at these for more in-depth information.

Generally speaking, if you graduate with a degree in sports science or a related area, you should be able to enter a job after university without having to do a postgraduate qualification. However, some people choose to continue studying either to become more specialised (for example, in biomechanics) or to improve their job prospects. Careers in research and academia normally require extra time spent in postgraduate study, either on an MSc course or a PhD.

At the end of their degree course, trainee podiatrists and physiotherapists will have undertaken sufficient study to qualify them to register with the Health Professions Council which, in turn, allows them to apply for work with such employers as the NHS. On-the-job training, however, is part of the job in both of these fields, as personal and professional development is essential to keep skills and knowledge of practice up to date.

For sports and exercise psychologists, gaining their undergraduate degree is just the first step on the career ladder. After graduating, they will need to undertake a further three years of postgraduate study, which will involve specialising in their chosen area, and carrying out supervised clinical placements, in order to reach chartered status. At this point, the job search normally begins.

What does a degree in these areas normally involve?

Again, the answer to this question will depend on what area of study you are hoping to go into. Below is a brief summary of the main degree subjects covered in this publication.

PODIATRY

Podiatry degrees cover everything you will need to know to enable you to practise as a podiatrist upon completion of the three-year course. This includes the anatomy, physiology, pathology, life sciences and body systems relating to the feet and lower limbs, as well as issues surrounding clinical practice, research, medicine and pharmacology. Often, certain subjects are studied alongside students in other disciplines, such as midwifery, pharmacology, nursing and physiotherapy, as this helps to introduce undergraduates to the multidisciplinary approach adopted in the healthcare professions as a whole.

Practical experience is vital in this degree, so students will find themselves working on patients, with supervision, to learn about how to conduct examinations, diagnoses, treatment and the use of appropriate equipment. The final year normally involves clinical placements in NHS settings such as hospital wards, outpatients and even in orthopaedic surgery.

PHYSIOTHERAPY

Physiotherapy students normally start off learning about the theory of practice. This involves studying aspects of anatomy, physiology, pathology and the musculoskeletal system. Other specialisms can be incorporated into this, including how health and illness affect the body, as well as neurological and cardio-respiratory problems. Some of the study will be combined with students on other related courses, particularly looking at aspects relating to ethics, the law and research. As with all healthcare courses, the chance to specialise is offered and you may be interested in taking up such options as acupuncture, sports medicine or hydrotherapy.

Practical experience is gained firstly by practising on your fellow students before you are allowed to try your skills out on the general public! Further into your training, you will be able to access clinical placements, often in each year of study.

SPORTS SCIENCE

Sports science involves looking (albeit probably in a more general way than physiotherapy and podiatry) at various biological areas of study, including anatomy, biomechanics, psychology, physiology, nutrition and metabolism, and relating them to how people perform physically. These biological subjects will be studied at a basic level at the start of any sports science degree, and will be looked at in more depth and detail in years two and three. Additionally, sports science undergraduates look at other aspects relating to the sporting arena, including management, business, technology, coaching and the analysis of performance.

SPORTS AND EXERCISE PSYCHOLOGY

All accredited psychology degrees cover the necessary theories and methods of psychology for you to attain the Graduate Basis for Registration (GBR), which is required by the British Psychological Society before you can progress further – if you so wish – with your training in this field. Courses usually last for three years, full time, though some four-year courses – with a year's work placement – are available. In the first year or two, students normally look at a wide range of psychological areas, such as cognitive psychology, use of statistics in analysis, research methods, language acquisition and development, and thinking and reasoning. In the final year, you will be able to specialise in your chosen topic, while carrying out a piece of research. Specialisms can range from the psychology of pain to looking at language disorders in children.

TEACHING METHODS

Most degree courses adopt a variety of different teaching methods: lectures, smaller group seminars, tutorials (often on a one-to-one basis), and practical workshops. This is something to consider when applying for courses as teaching methods can vary. Equally assessment methods differ between universities. Some of the more traditional institutions rely on final examinations, while others assess students through either continuous assessment or a mixture of final exams and coursework.

ENTRY REQUIREMENTS

Which subjects?

While you don't need to have all three sciences at A level for sports science and related areas, admissions tutors normally prefer at least one out of chemistry, physics, biology or maths, and some will not accept physical education as a substitute for one of these, although it is welcomed as an additional A level. Psychology A level is not a prerequisite for a psychology degree, although it can be a useful introduction to the subject area. Normally a combination of good results in academic A level subjects are accepted, but sometimes general studies is not considered worthy of an offer.

Competition for places on UK sports science and related courses is very tough and it is thought that it will become even fiercer with interest in these areas peaking as a result of the London 2012 Olympics. Therefore, it is not uncommon for admissions tutors to request high grades or UCAS Tariff points. Check with each institution for their entry requirements. Tutors may also take GCSE grades into account as another way to filter the growing number of straight-A students.

TOP TIP

Don't be afraid to pick up the phone – university admissions offices welcome enquiries directly from students, rather than careers officers on your behalf. It shows you're genuinely interested and committed to your career early on.

Applicant journey

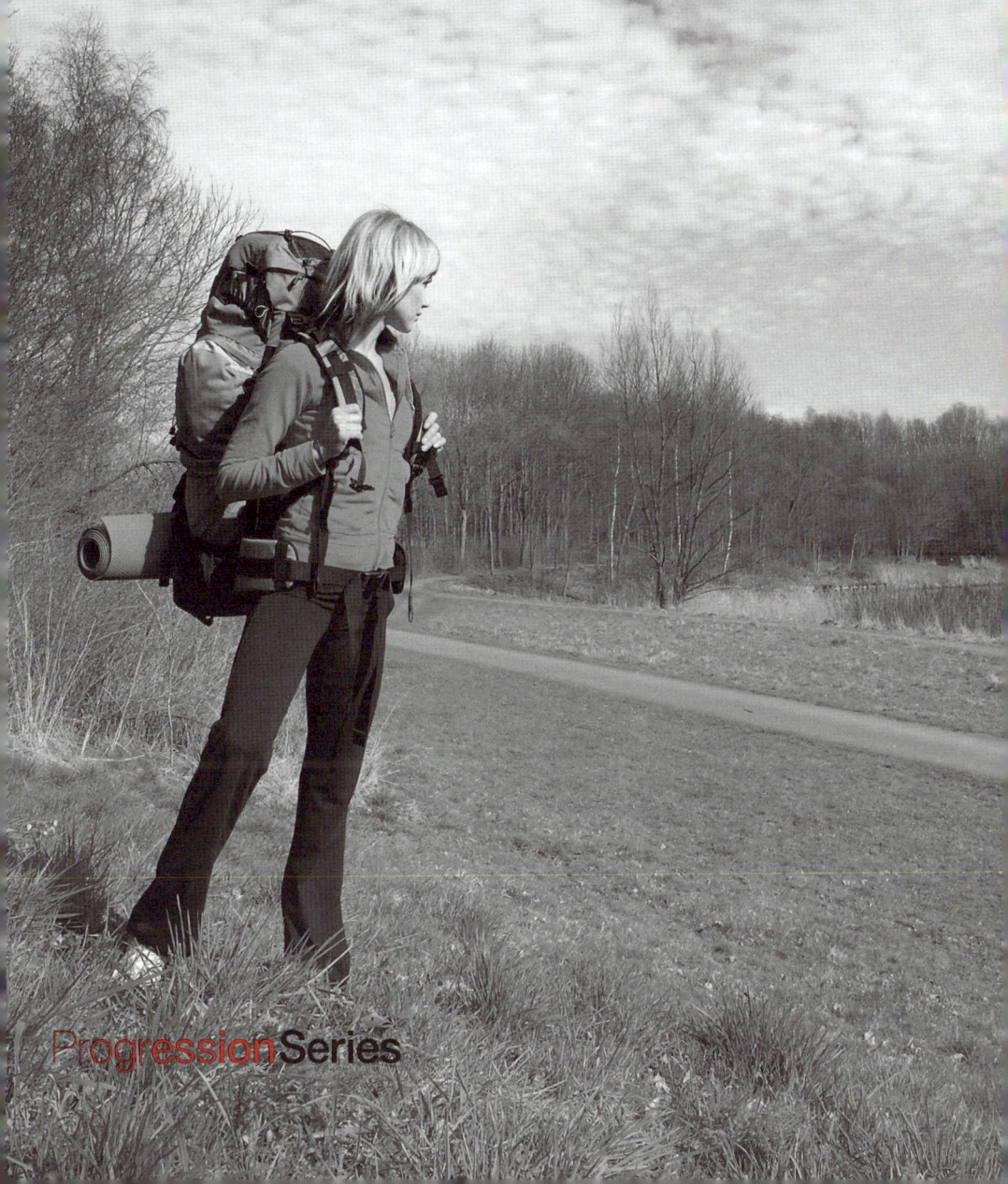

SIX EASY STEPS TO UNIVERSITY AND COLLEGE

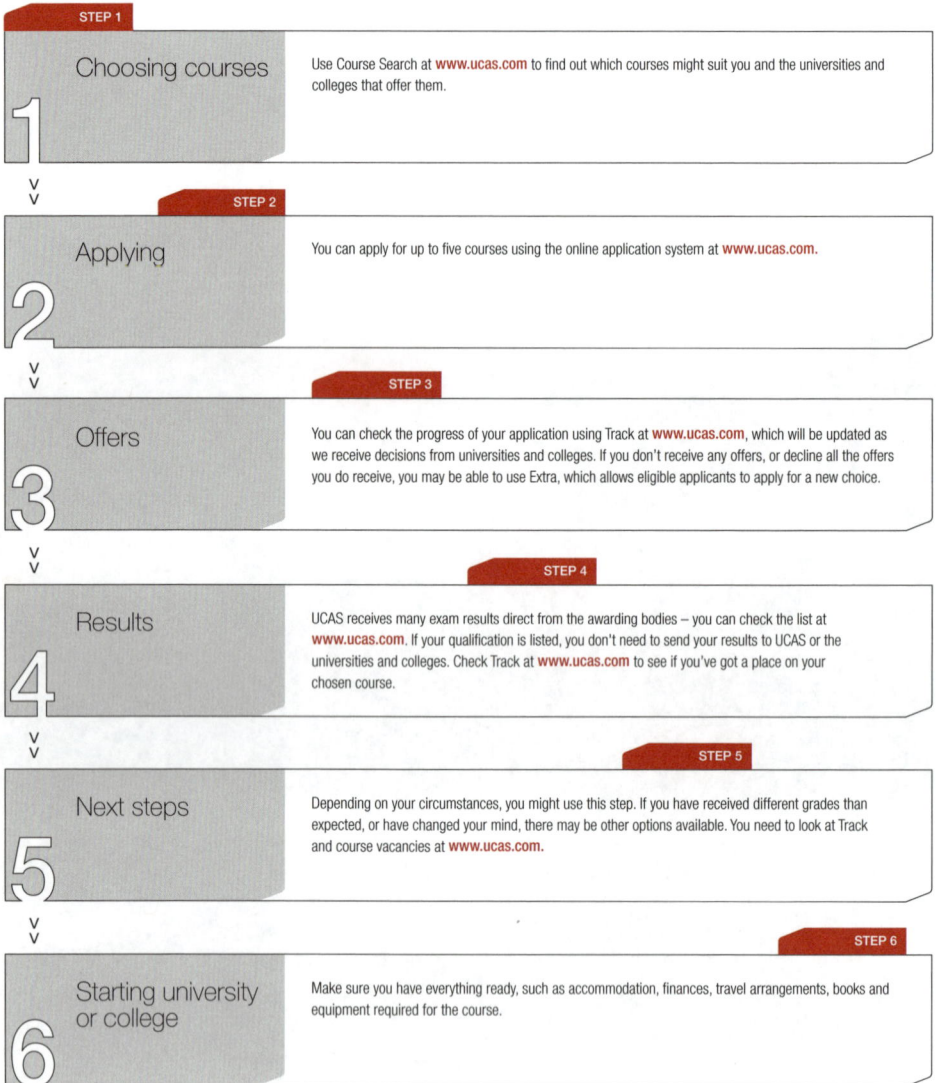

STEP 1

1

Choosing courses

Use Course Search at **www.ucas.com** to find out which courses might suit you and the universities and colleges that offer them.

STEP 2

2

Applying

You can apply for up to five courses using the online application system at **www.ucas.com.**

STEP 3

3

Offers

You can check the progress of your application using Track at **www.ucas.com**, which will be updated as we receive decisions from universities and colleges. If you don't receive any offers, or decline all the offers you do receive, you may be able to use Extra, which allows eligible applicants to apply for a new choice.

STEP 4

4

Results

UCAS receives many exam results direct from the awarding bodies – you can check the list at **www.ucas.com**. If your qualification is listed, you don't need to send your results to UCAS or the universities and colleges. Check Track at **www.ucas.com** to see if you've got a place on your chosen course.

STEP 5

5

Next steps

Depending on your circumstances, you might use this step. If you have received different grades than expected, or have changed your mind, there may be other options available. You need to look at Track and course vacancies at **www.ucas.com.**

STEP 6

6

Starting university or college

Make sure you have everything ready, such as accommodation, finances, travel arrangements, books and equipment required for the course.

1 Choosing courses

Step 1 – Planning your application for sports science and physiotherapy

Planning your application is the start of your journey to finding a place at a university or college.

This section will help you decide what course to study and how to choose a university or college where you'll enjoy living and studying. Find out about qualifications, degree options, how they'll assess you, and coping with the costs of higher education.

1 Choosing courses

Choosing courses

USE COURSE SEARCH AT WWW.UCAS.COM TO FIND OUT WHICH COURSES MIGHT SUIT YOU, AND THE UNIVERSITIES AND COLLEGES THAT OFFER THEM

Start thinking about what you want to study and where you want to go. Read the section on 'Finding a course' (page 67), and see what courses are available where in the chapter on 'Courses' (page 115). Check the entry requirements required for each course meet your academic expectations.

Use the UCAS website – www.ucas.com has lots of advice on how to find a course. Go to the students' section of the website for the best advice or go straight to Course Search to see all the courses available through UCAS. See the section on Entry Profiles on page 68-69 which explains what they are and how to find them on our website.

Watch UCAStv – at www.ucas.tv there are videos on 'how to choose your course', 'attending events' as well as case studies and video diaries from students talking about their experience of finding a course at university or college.

Attend UCAS conventions – UCAS conventions are held throughout the country. Universities and colleges have exhibition stands where their staff offer information about their courses and institutions. Details of when the conventions are happening are shown at **www.ucas.com/students/exhibitions.**

Look at the prospectuses – Universities and colleges have prospectuses and course-specific leaflets on their undergraduate courses. Your school or college library may have copies or go to the university's website to download a copy or you can ask them to send one to you.

Go to university open days – most institutions offer open days to anyone who wants to attend. See the institution information pages on Course Search and the UCAS/COA Open Days publication (see page 109) for information on when they are taking place.

League tables – these can be helpful but bear in mind that they attempt to rank institutions in an overall order reflecting the views of those that produce them. They may not reflect your views and needs.

Do your research – speak and refer to as many trusted sources as you can find. The section on 'Which area?' on pages 16-35 will help you identify the different areas of sports science and physiotherapy you might want to enter.

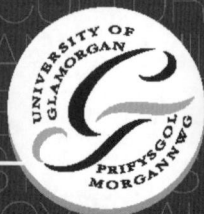

1

Choosing courses

Finding a course

Through UCAS you can apply to five courses in total. How do you find out more information to make an informed decision?

How do you narrow down your choices to five? First of all, look up course details in this book or online on **www.ucas.com**. This will give you an idea of the full range of courses and topics on offer. You'll quickly be able to eliminate institutions that don't offer the right course, or you can choose a 'hit list' of institutions first, and then see what they have to offer.

Once you've made a short(er) list, read the university and college Entry Profiles (see the next page) to find out what particular courses offer. You can then follow this up by looking at university or college websites, and generally finding out as much as you can about the course, department and institution. Don't be afraid to contact them to ask for more information, request their prospectus or arrange an open day visit.

UCAS WEBSITE – www.ucas.com

Whether you want advice about applying to higher education, to check out what courses are available, to find out what qualifications you need, or to monitor the status of your application, **www.ucas.com** is a great place to start. The UCAS website is one of the most popular websites in the UK and the most heavily used educational one, with over 1.5 million unique users a month. It is popular for good reason. From it, you can use Course Search as a quick and easy way to find out more about the courses you are interested in, including the vital code information you will need to include in your application later on. From Course Search, you can link to the websites of the universities and colleges in the UCAS system. Once you've applied through UCAS, you can use Track to check the progress of your application, including any decisions from universities or colleges, and you can make replies to your offers online.

1 Choosing courses

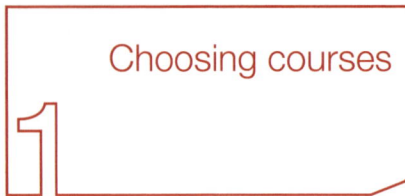

Entry Profiles

WHAT ARE THEY?

Entry Profiles give potential applicants to higher education specific information to help them make informed decisions about the courses they apply for. Detailed knowledge about the course, formal entry requirements and the qualities and experiences institutions are looking for in their applicants can help ensure that every applicant finds their way onto the right course. Entry Profiles are published on the UCAS website and can be reached using Course Search. They are available for all potential applicants and their advisers to see as they start making important decisions about where to apply. All course providers are asked to contribute Entry Profiles for the UCAS Course Search facility.

WHY USE THEM?

Courses can vary at different universities and colleges, even when they have the same name. Differences in course content, structure, optional modules, and the department's approach to teaching and learning can make the experience of studying any subject very different for students at different institutions, even before the size and location of the institution are taken into account.

It is important that you are fully informed about the courses and the institutions offering them before you apply, and that you know what academic qualifications and personal qualities are being sought in an applicant. Then you can avoid mistakes and make fully informed choices.

HOW DO I USE THE ENTRY PROFILES?

- When you find courses that interest you, search for the Entry Profile through the Course Search at www.ucas.com. Look for the symbol EP after the course title on the results page. This tells you that it has a complete Entry Profile.
- Courses without the EP symbol have academic entry requirements only.

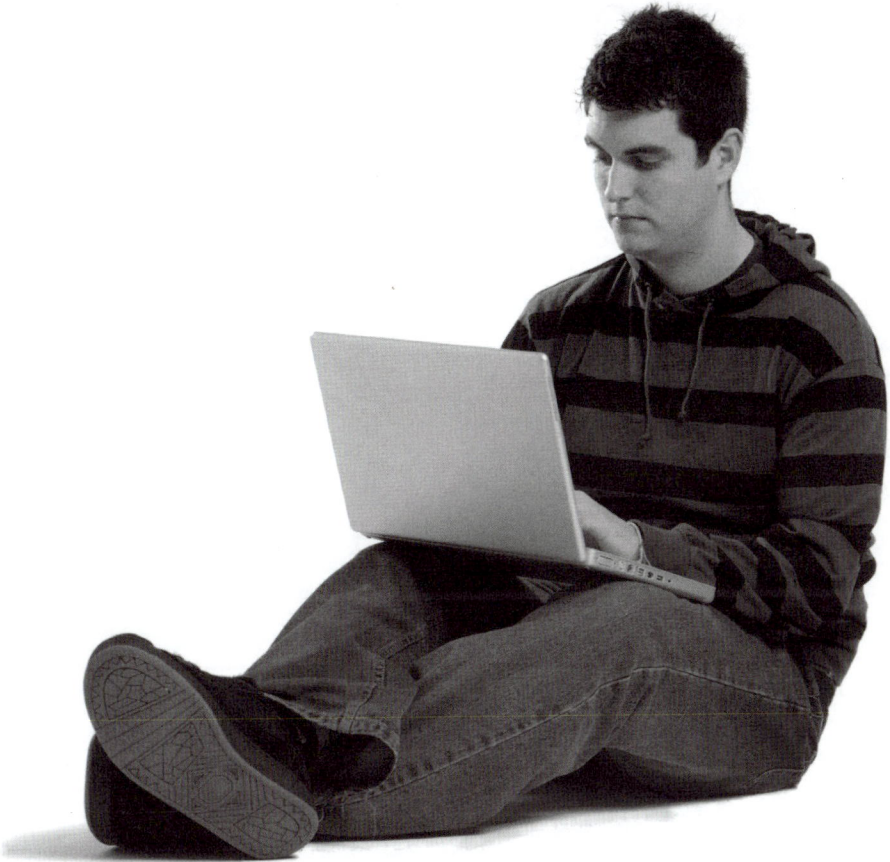

1

Choosing courses

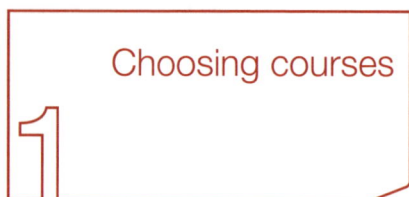

Choosing your institution

Different people look for different things from their university or college course, but the checklist on the next page sets out the kinds of factors all prospective students should consider when choosing their university. Keep this list in mind on open days, when talking to friends about their experiences at various universities and colleges, or while reading prospectuses and websites.

WHAT TO CONSIDER WHEN CHOOSING YOUR SPORTS SCIENCE AND PHYSIOTHERAPY COURSE

Location	Do you want to stay close to home. Would you prefer to study at a city or campus university or college?
Grades required	Use the Course Search facility on the UCAS website, www.ucas.com, to view entry requirements for courses you are interested in. Also, check out the university or college website or call up the admissions office. Some institutions specify 'grades' required, eg AAB, while others specify 'points' required, eg 340. If they ask for points, it means they're using the UCAS Tariff system, which basically awards points to different types and levels of qualification. For example, an A grade at A level = 120 points; a B grade at A level = 100 points. The full Tariff tables are available on pages 94–99 and at www.ucas.com.
Employer links	Ask the course tutor or department about links with employers, especially for placements or work experience.
Graduate prospects	Ask the careers office for their list of graduate 'destinations'.
Cost	Ask the admissions office about variable tuition fees and financial assistance.
Sports science and physiotherapy or non-sports science and physiotherapy degree?	Is there another subject that you enjoy, that you could study first, that might actually help give you an edge in employers' eyes?
Degree type	Do you want to study sports science and physiotherapy on its own ('single' honours degree) or 50/50 with another subject ('joint') or as one of a few subjects ('combined' degree)? If you opt for a joint or combined course, check that you won't need to do a conversion course to pursue your chosen career.
Teaching style	How many lectures per week, amount of tutorial or one-to-one work, etc?
Course assessment	Can you see yourself writing essays throughout the year?
Facilities for students	Check out the library and sporting facilities, and find out if there is a careers adviser dedicated to your subject.
'Fit'	Even if all the above criteria stack up, this one relies on gut feel – go and visit the institution if you can and see if it's 'you'.

1

Choosing courses

How will they choose you?

Most admissions departments will have different entry criteria, so make sure that you check prospectuses, websites and all other materials thoroughly before you apply. Even better, why not give them a call and discuss it with them directly? Not only will it leave you better prepared to submit a targeted application, but it will also demonstrate that you're self-motivated.

It's unlikely that you'll have to sit an entry test. This means that if there is an interview (and in many cases there will be) it is particularly important.

THE INTERVIEW

Talk to someone who has been – or is currently – on the course that you are applying for. What was their interview like? What kinds of questions were they asked? Be prepared and if possible do a mock interview with a friend, relative or school careers adviser before you go for the real thing.

Choosing courses

1

The cost of higher education

As a student, you will have to pay for two things:

- tuition fees for your course
- living costs, such as rent, food, books, transport and entertainment.

If that sounds expensive, don't worry. You can get financial help from the Government in the form of loans and grants.

FEES

The amount of tuition fees you have to pay, and the financial assistance you may be entitled to, depends on:

- where you live
- where you want to study
- what you want to study
- your financial circumstances.

STUDENT LOANS, GRANTS AND BURSARIES

The purpose of a student loan is to help cover the costs of your tuition fees and basic living (rent, bills, food etc). Many other kinds of loan are available to students while they are studying at university or college. Depending on the source of the loan, the interest rate can have a severe impact upon the overall debt at the end of your degree. However, a student loan (or student maintenance loan as it is sometimes known) only takes inflation into account, so the overall amount you owe will only be slightly higher than the figure borrowed. Maintenance loans are available to all citizens who satisfy UK residency requirements.

Remember that a student loan is not a grant: you do have to pay it back once you have left university and are earning over £15,000 a year.

In addition, there are non-repayable grants and bursaries available, depending on your circumstances and the courses and institutions to which you are applying.

USEFUL WEBSITES

There is lots of information available about student finance. Listed below are some websites you may find useful:

UCAS
www.ucas.com/students/studentfinance

National Union of Students
www.nus.org.uk/money

If your family lives in England, you should visit
www.direct.gov.uk/studentfinance.

If your family lives in Wales, you should visit
www.studentfinancewales.co.uk
www.cyllidmyfyrwyrcymru.co.uk.

If your family lives in Northern Ireland, you should visit
www.studentfinanceni.co.uk.

If your family lives in Scotland, you should visit
www.saas.gov.uk.

Disabled Students' Allowance
If you have a disablilty or specific learning difficulty you may be able to apply for a Disabled Students' Allowance. To find out more go to the websites above and search on Disabled Student.

Childcare Grant
This is available to students who have dependent children and a low household income. This includes students who are lone parents and students who are married to, or the partners of, other students.

NHS Funding
It is possible for students on NHS funded degrees to apply for NHS busaries.
www.nhsstudentgrants.co.uk/.

TOP TIP

Before you choose your institution, make sure you find out about the bursaries they offer. Some are likely to be more generous than others, and this may make the difference between a financially comfortable or uncomfortable time.

1 Choosing courses

International students

APPLYING TO STUDY IN THE UK

Deciding to go to university or college in the UK is very exciting. You need to think about what course to do, where to study, and how much it will cost. The decisions you make can have a huge effect on your future but UCAS is here to help.

What is UCAS?

UCAS is the organisation that manages applications to full-time undergraduate courses in the UK. All the UK universities and many colleges use us. We are respected around the world and you can access our website 24 hours a day, seven days a week at **www.ucas.com**.

Whatever your age or qualifications, if you want to apply for any of the 50,000 courses listed at over 300 universities and colleges on the UCAS website, you must apply through UCAS at **www.ucas.com**. If you are unsure, your school, college, adviser, or local British Council office will be able to help. Further advice and a video guide for international students can be found on the non-UK section of the UCAS website at **www.ucas.com/students/nonukstudents**.

What is Apply?

Apply is our secure online application system that you can use anytime and anywhere, giving you the flexibility to fill in your application when it suits you. Each time you log in, you can enter more information and take as long as you wish to change and complete it. Using Apply is the fastest and most efficient method of applying, but students with limited or no internet access should contact the UCAS Customer Service Unit on +44 (0)870 11 222 11 for advice on what to do. By applying through UCAS, you are able to use the one application for up to five choices.

Students may apply on their own or through their school, college, adviser, or local British Council if they are registered with UCAS to use Apply. If you choose to use an education agent's services, check with the British Council to see if they hold a list of certificated or registered agents in your country. Check also on any charges you may need to pay. UCAS charges only the application fee (see below) but agents may charge for additional services.

How much will my application cost?

If you choose to apply to more than one course, university or college you need to pay UCAS £19 GBP when you apply. If you only apply to one course at one university or college, you pay UCAS £9 GBP.

WHAT LEVEL OF ENGLISH?

UCAS provides a list of English language qualifications and grades that are acceptable to most UK universities and colleges, however you are advised to contact the institutions directly as each have their own entry requirement in English. For more information go to **www.ucas.com/students/nonukstudents/englangprof**.

INTERNATIONAL STUDENT FEES

If you study in the UK, your fee status (whether you pay full-cost fees or a subsidised fee rate) will be decided by the UK university or college you plan to attend. Before you decide which university or college to attend, you need to be absolutely certain that you can pay the full cost of:

- your tuition fees (the amount is set by universities and colleges, so contact them for more information – visit their websites where many list their fees)
- the everyday living expenses for you and your family for the whole time that you are in the UK, including accommodation, food, heat, light, clothes, travel
- books and equipment for your course
- travel to and from your country.

You must include everything when you work out how much it will cost. You can get information to help you do this accurately from the international offices at universities and colleges, UKCISA (UK Council for International Student Affairs) and the British Council. There is a useful website tool to help you manage your money at university – **www.studentcalculator.org.uk**.

Scholarships and bursaries are offered at some universities and colleges and you should contact them for more information. In addition, you should check with your local British Council for additional scholarships available to students from your country who want to study in the UK.

LEGAL DOCUMENTS YOU WILL NEED

As you prepare to study in the UK, it is very important to think about the legal documents you will need to enter the country.

Everyone who comes to study in the UK needs a valid passport. If you do not have one, you should apply for one as soon as possible. People from certain countries also need visas before they come into the UK. They are known as 'visa nationals'. You can check if you require a visa to travel to the UK by visiting the UK Border Agency website and selecting "Studying in the UK". So, please check the UK Border Agency website at **www.ukba.homeoffice.gov.uk** for the most up-to-date guidance and information about the United Kingdom's visa requirements.

When you apply for your visa you need to make sure you have the following documents:

- A visa letter from the university or college where you are going to study or a Confirmation of Acceptance for Study (CAS) number. The university or college must be on the UKBA Register of Sponsors.
- A valid passport.
- Evidence that you have enough money to pay for your course and living costs.
- Certificates for all qualifications you have that are relevant to the course you have been accepted for and for any English language qualifications.

You will also have to give your biometric data.

Do check for further information from your local British Embassy or High Commission. Guidance information for international students is also available from UKCISA and from UKBA.

ADDITIONAL RESOURCES

There are a number of organisations that can provide further guidance and information to you as you prepare to study in the UK:

- British Council
  www.britishcouncil.org
- Education UK (British Council website dealing with educational matters)
  www.educationuk.org
- English UK (British Council accredited website listing English language courses in the UK)
  www.englishuk.com
- UK Border Agency (provides information on visa requirements and applications)
  www.ukba.homeoffice.gov.uk
- UKCISA (UK Council for International Student Affairs)
  www.ukcisa.org.uk
- BUILA (British Universities, International Liaison Association)
  www.buila.ac.uk
- DIUS (Department for Innovation, Universities and Skills)
  www.dius.gov.uk

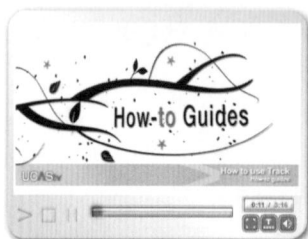

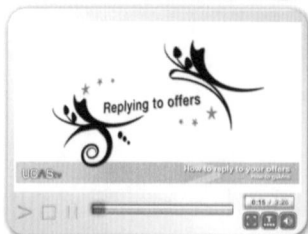

Applying

2

Step 2 – Applying

Apply for up to five courses using the UCAS online application system at **www.ucas.com**

WHEN TO APPLY

Make a note of these important dates for your diary.

- **Early September 2009**
  Opening date for receiving applications.
- **15 October 2009**
  Application deadline for the receipt at UCAS of applications for all medicine, dentistry, veterinary medicine and veterinary science courses and for all courses at the universities of Oxford and Cambridge.
- **15 January 2010**
  Application deadline for the receipt at UCAS of applications for all courses except those listed above with a 15 October deadline.

- **25 February 2010**
  Start of Extra.
- **30 June 2010**
  Final deadline for all applications, including those from outside the UK and EU. Any applications we receive after this date go directly into Clearing.
- **20 September 2010**
  Last date for Clearing applications.

Don't forget…

Universities and colleges guarantee to consider your application if we receive it by the appropriate deadline. If you send it in after the deadline, but by 30 June 2010, universities and colleges will consider it if they want to make more offers.

Applying

2

How to apply

You apply online at **www.ucas.com** through Apply – a secure, web-based application service that is designed for all our applicants, whether they are applying through a UCAS-registered centre or as an individual, anywhere in the world. Apply is:

- easy to access – all you need is an internet connection
- easy to use – you don't have to complete your application all in one go: you can save the sections as you complete them and come back to it later
- easy to monitor – once you've applied, you can use Track to check the progress of your application, including any decisions from universities or colleges. You can also reply to your offers using Track
- watch the UCAStv guide to applying through UCAS at **www.ucas.tv**.

DEFERRED ENTRY

If you want to apply for deferred entry in 2011, perhaps because you want to take a year out between school or college and higher education, you should check that the university or college will accept a deferred entry application. Occasionally, tutors are not happy to accept students who take a gap year, because it interrupts the flow of their learning. If you apply for deferred entry, you must meet the conditions of any offers by 31 August 2010. If you accept a place for 2011 entry and then change your mind, you cannot reapply through us in the 2011 entry cycle unless you withdraw your original application.

INVISIBILITY OF CHOICES

Universities and colleges cannot see details of the other choices on your application until you reply to any offers or you have not been successful at any of your choices.

You can only submit one UCAS application in each year's application cycle.

APPLYING THROUGH YOUR SCHOOL OR COLLEGE

1 GET SCHOOL OR COLLEGE 'BUZZWORD'

Ask your UCAS application coordinator (may be your sixth form tutor) for your school or college UCAS 'buzzword'. This is a password for the school or college.

2 REGISTER

Go to **www.ucas.com/students/apply** and click on **Register/Log in** to use **Apply** and then **Register**. After you have entered your registration details, the online system will automatically generate a username for you, but you'll have to come up with a password and answers to security questions.

3 COMPLETE SIX SECTIONS

Complete the sections of the application. To access any section, click on the section name at the top of the screen and follow the instructions. The sections are:

Personal details – contact details, residential status, disability status

Additional information – only UK applicants need to complete this section

Choices – which courses you'd like to apply for

Education – your education to date

Employment – for example, work experience, holiday jobs

Personal statement – page 84.

4 PASS TO REFEREE

Once you've completed all the sections, send your application electronically to your referee (normally your form tutor). They'll check it, approve it and add their reference to it, and will then send it to UCAS on your behalf.

USEFUL INFORMATION ABOUT APPLY

- Important details like date of birth and course codes will be checked by Apply. It will alert you if they are not valid.
- The text for your personal statement and reference can be copied and pasted into your application.
- You can change your application at any time before it is completed and sent to UCAS.
- You can print and preview your application at any time.
- Your application will normally be processed at UCAS within one working day.
- Your school, college or centre can choose different payment methods. For example, they may want us to bill them, or you may be able to pay online by debit or credit card.

NOT APPLYING THROUGH A SCHOOL OR COLLEGE

For example, if you are not currently studying – you can follow the same steps, but, as you can't supply a 'buzzword', you'll just be asked a few extra questions to check you are eligible to apply, and you'll have to supply a reference from someone who knows you well enough to comment on your suitability for higher education. Guidance on choosing a suitable referee is available in Apply and on the UCAS website. If you are not applying through a school, college or other UCAS-registered centre, you should apply online and pay by debit or credit card.

If you have recently left school or college you can ask them to supply your reference online.

wondering how much higher education costs?

need information about variable fees, grants and student loans?

Visit www.ucas.com/studentfinance and discover everything you need to know about student money matters.

With access to up-to-date information on bursaries, scholarships and variable fees, plus our online budget calculator. Visit us today and get the full picture.

UCAS helping students into higher education www.ucas.com/studentfinance

Applying

2

Making your application

We want this to run smoothly for you and we also want to process your application as quickly as possible. You can help us to do this by remembering to do the following:

- check the closing dates for applications – see page 79
- start early and allow plenty of time for completing your application – including enough time for your referee to complete the reference section
- read the instructions carefully before you start
- consider what each question is actually asking for
- ask a teacher, parent, friend or careers adviser to review your draft application – particularly the personal statement
- pay special attention to questions that ask you about your interests and experience

- if you have extra information that will not fit on your application, send it direct to your chosen universities or colleges after we have sent you your Welcome letter with your Personal ID – don't send it to us
- keep a copy of the final version of your application, in case you are asked questions on it at an interview.

Applying

2

The personal statement

Next to choosing your courses, this section of your application will take up most of your time. It is of immense importance as many colleges and universities rely solely on the information in the UCAS application, rather than interviews and admissions tests, when selecting students. The personal statement can be the deciding factor in whether or not they offer you a place. If it is an institution that interviews, it could be the deciding factor in whether you get called for interview.

Keep a copy of your personal statement – if you are called for interview, you will almost certainly be asked questions based on it.

Tutors will look carefully at your exam results, actual and predicted, your referee's statement and your own personal statement. Remember, they are looking for reasons to offer you a place – try to give them every opportunity to do so!

A SALES DOCUMENT

The personal statement is your opportunity to sell yourself, so do so. The university or college admissions tutor who reads your personal statement wants to get a rounded picture of you to decide whether you will make an interesting member of the university or college both academically and socially. They want to know more about you than the subjects you are studying at school.

HOW TO IMPRESS

Don't be put off by the blank space. The secret is to cover key areas that admissions tutors always look for. Include things like hobbies and work experience, especially if they are linked in some way to the type of course you are applying for. You could talk about your career plans and interesting things you might have done outside the classroom. Have you belonged to sports teams or orchestras or held positions of responsibility? Maybe you've been a school play stalwart or been involved in community activities. If you left full-time education a while ago, talk about the work you have done and the skills you have gathered or how you have juggled bringing up a family – that is evidence of time management skills. Whoever you are, make sure you explain what appeals to you about the course you are applying for.

A lot of the interview will be based on information supplied on your application – especially your **personal statement.** Visit www.ucas.tv to view the video to help guide you through the process, and address the most common fears and concerns about writing a personal statement.

WHAT ADMISSIONS TUTORS LOOK FOR

- Your reasons for wanting to take this course.
- Your communication skills – how you express yourself in the personal statement.
- Relevant experience – experience that's related to your choice of course.
- Evidence of your interest in this field.
- Evidence of your teamwork.
- Evidence of your skills, for example, IT skills, people skills, debating and public speaking.
- Other activities that show your dedication and ability to apply yourself.

WHAT TO TELL THEM

- Why you want to do this subject.
- What experience you already have in this field – for example work experience, school projects, hobbies, voluntary work.
- The skills and qualities you have as a person that would make you a good student, for example anything that shows your dedication, communication ability, academic achievement, initiative.
- Anything that shows you can knuckle down and apply yourself, for example running a marathon, raising money for charity.
- If you're taking a gap year, why and (if possible) what you're going to do during it.
- About your other interests and activities away from studying – to show you're a 'rounded' person.

WORK EXPERIENCE

How much does it count? Ask any admissions tutor or recruiter about the importance of work experience on a candidate's application and they'll all agree – work experience shows a real, rather than theoretical, interest in your chosen field. An absence of work experience suggests questionable commitment to your choice of career.

Work experience will not only give you a real insight into the work of a sports scientist or physiotherapist, it will also give you valuable examples of the skills you have to offer.

Work experience is especially useful to help you find out what you want to do. Since sports science and related areas are involved in people-centred professions, work experience in a setting where you are dealing with a variety of individuals could help you to find out early on if it a career in this area really is for you. Try to ask sports and other health charities for advice and opportunities as well as contacting your local NHS Trust, city or county council and schools. Additionally, if sports science is more your thing, it goes without saying that participation in sports will be looked for so make the most of any activities you enjoy, from dancing and darts to swimming and shot-put.

Work experience can add impact to your personal statement by showing that you understand what you're getting into, and that you have explored the area in a practical way over a period of time.

Make sure you find out about work experience routes for the dedicated A level student, including taster days and introductory courses offered by universities and colleges, volunteering at your local leisure centre, community centre or hospital.

Offers

3

Step 3 – Offers

Once we have sent your application to your chosen universities and colleges, they will all consider it independently and tell us whether or not they can offer you a place. Some universities and colleges will take longer to make decisions than others. You may be asked to attend an interview, sit an additional test or provide a piece of work such as an essay before a decision can be made.

You may or may not be called for an interview as part of the selection process. Many institutions prefer not to interview people, as it's a very subjective and time-consuming process. However, some interview candidates as a matter of course, and others interview to clarify some aspect of a candidate's application – for example, if you're an international student in the UK to check your communication skills, or if your grades are borderline.

If you are called for interview, the key areas they are likely to cover will be:

- evidence of your academic ability
- your capacity to study hard
- your commitment to a sports science or physiotherapy career, best shown by work experience and sports involvement
- your logic and reasoning ability.

A lot of the interview will be based on information supplied on your application – especially your **personal statement** – see pages 84-86 for tips about the personal statement.

Each time a university or college makes a decision about your application we record it and let you know. You can check the progress of your application using Track at **www.ucas.com**. This is our secure online service which gives you access to your application using the same username and password you used when you applied. You can use it to find out if you have been invited for interview or need to provide an additional piece of work, as well as check to see if you have received any offers.

Find out more about how to use Track in the UCAStv video guide at **www.ucas.tv**.

Types of offer

Universities and colleges can make two types of offer: conditional or unconditional. If they want you to pass your exams before they can accept you, they will make a conditional offer. The conditions of the offer may specify the number of UCAS Tariff points, for example 200 points from three A levels, or the grades for your A levels, such as B in English and C in history.

If they want to offer you a place and you already have all the necessary qualifications, they will make you an unconditional offer. This means that if you accept this offer you have a definite place.

However, for either type of offer there may be some non-academic requirements:

- For courses that involve contact with children and vulnerable adults you may need to have criminal record checks and ISA registration before you can start the course.
- For health courses you will need to have a health check.
- For students who are not resident in either the UK or the EU, there may be some financial conditions to meet.

Replying to offers

When you have received decisions for all your choices, you must decide what you want to accept and you do this by using Track. You will be given a deadline by which to decide what to accept.

You can accept up to two offers. If you accept a conditional offer as your firm or preferred choice, you may accept another offer as an insurance or back-up choice. You may accept an unconditional or conditional offer as your insurance choice. If you accept an unconditional offer as your firm or preferred choice, you cannot accept another offer and you will go straight to step 6 of your applicant journey (see page 105).

When you accept your firm and, if permitted, insurance choice, you must turn down all your other offers.

If you turn down all your offers, you may be able to apply for further courses using Extra (page 90). If you are not eligible to use Extra, you can contact universities and colleges with vacancies in Clearing (page 102). For more information and advice about replying to your offers, watch the UCAStv video guide at **www.ucas.tv**.

What if you have no offers?

If you have applied through UCAS and are not holding any offers, you may be able to add more choices, if you have not used all five choices, or apply through Extra for another course.

If you are not eligible for Extra, you can contact universities and colleges with vacancies in Clearing from mid-July 2010 (page 102).

3 | Offers

Extra

Extra allows you to make additional choices, one at a time, without having to wait for Clearing in July. It is completely optional and free, and is designed to encourage you to continue researching and choosing courses if you need to. The courses available through Extra will be highlighted on Course Search, at **www.ucas.com**.

Who is eligible?

You will be eligible for Extra if you have already made five choices and:

- you have had unsuccessful or withdrawal decisions from all five of your choices, or
- you have cancelled your outstanding choices and hold no offers, or
- you have received decisions from all five choices and have declined all offers made to you.

How does it work?

We contact you and explain what to do if you are eligible for Extra. If you are eligible you should:

- see a special Extra button on your Track screen
- check on Course Search for courses that are available through Extra; they are shown by the symbol X after the course title.
- choose one that you would like to apply for and enter the details on your Track screen.

When you have chosen a course, a copy of your application will be sent to the university or college.

What happens next?

We give universities and colleges 21 days to consider your Extra application. During this time, you cannot be considered by another university or college. After 21 days you can refer yourself to a different university or college if you wish, but it is a good idea to ring the one currently considering you before doing so. If you are made an offer, you can choose whether or not to accept it.

If you are currently studying for examinations, any offer that you receive is likely to be an offer conditional on exam grades. If you decide to accept a conditional offer, you will not be able to take any further part in Extra.

If you already have your examination results, it is possible that a university or college may make an unconditional offer.

If you accept an unconditional offer, you will be placed. You cannot then apply to any other universities or colleges in Extra.

If you decide to decline the offer, or the university or college decides they cannot make you an offer, you will be given another opportunity to use Extra, time permitting. Your Extra button on Track will be reactivated.

Once you have accepted an offer in Extra, you are committed to it in the same way as you would be with an offer through the main UCAS system. Conditional offers made through Extra will be treated in the same way as other conditional offers, when your examination results become available.

If your results do not meet the conditions and the university or college decides that they cannot confirm your Extra offer, you will automatically become eligible for Clearing if it is too late for you to be considered by another university or college in Extra.

If you are unsuccessful, decline an offer, or do not receive an offer, or 21 days has elapsed since choosing a course through Extra, you can use Extra to apply for another course.

From 1 October – 30 June

Applicants informed as they become eligible for Extra.

From 25 February – early July

The Extra service is available to eligible applicants through Track at **www.ucas.com**.

Advice

Do some careful research and seek guidance on your Extra choice of university or college and course. If you applied to high-demand courses and institutions in your original application and were unsuccessful, you could consider related or alternative subjects or perhaps apply for the subject you want in combination with another. Your teachers or careers advisers or the universities and colleges themselves can provide useful guidance. Entry Profiles, which appear with most courses listed on Course Search, are another important source of information. Be flexible, that is the key to success. But you are the only one who knows how flexible you are prepared to be. Remember that even if you decide to take a degree course other than sports science or physiotherapy, you may be able to take an alternative route into the profession.

Visit **www.ucas.tv** to watch the video guide on how to use Extra.

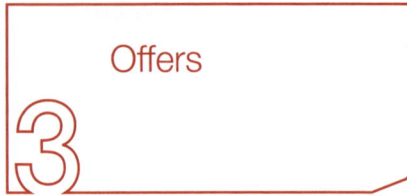

Offers

3

The Tariff

Admission to higher education courses is generally dependent upon an individual's achievement in level 3 qualifications, such as GCE A levels. Did you know that there are currently over 3,000 level 3 qualifications available in the UK alone?

As if the number of qualifications available was not confusing enough, different qualifications can have different grading structures (alphabetical, numerical or a mixture of both). Finding out what qualifications are needed for different higher education courses can be very confusing.

The UCAS Tariff is the system for allocating points to qualifications used for entry to HE. It allows students to use a range of different qualifications to help secure a place on an undergraduate course.

Universities and colleges use the UCAS Tariff to make comparisons between applicants with different qualifications. Tariff points are often used in entry requirements, although other factors are often taken into account. Entry Profiles provide a fuller picture of what admissions tutors are seeking.

The tables on the following pages show the qualifications covered by the UCAS Tariff. There may have been changes to these tables since this book was printed. You should visit www.ucas.com to view the most up-to-date tables.

FURTHER INFORMATION?

Although Tariff points can be accumulated in a variety of ways, not all of these will necessarily be acceptable for entry to a particular HE course. The achievement of a points score therefore does not give an automatic entitlement to entry, and many other factors are taken into account in the admissions process.

The Course Search facility at www.ucas.com is the best source of reference to find out what qualifications are acceptable for entry to specific courses. Updates to the Tariff, including details on how new qualifications are added, can be found at www.ucas.com/students/ucas_tariff/.

HOW DOES THE TARIFF WORK?

- Students can collect Tariff points from a range of different qualifications, eg GCE A level with BTEC Nationals.
- There is no ceiling to the number of points that can be accumulated.
- There is no double counting. Certain qualifications within the Tariff build on qualifications in the same subject. In these cases only the qualification with the higher Tariff score will be counted. This principle applies to:
    - GCE Advanced Subsidiary level and GCE Advanced level
    - Scottish Highers and Advanced Highers
    - Key Skills at level 2, 3 and 4
    - Speech, drama and music awards at grades 6, 7 and 8.
- Tariff points for the Advanced Diploma come from the Progression Diploma score plus the relevant Additional and Specialist Learning (ASL) Tariff points. Please see the appropriate qualification in the Tariff tables to calculate the ASL score.
- The Extended Project Tariff points are included within the Tariff points for Progression and Advanced Diplomas. Extended Project points represented in the Tariff only count when the qualification is taken outside of these Diplomas.
- Where the Tariff tables refer to specific awarding bodies, only qualifications from these awarding bodies attract Tariff points. Qualifications with a similar title, but from a different qualification awarding body do not attract Tariff points.

HOW DO UNIVERSITIES AND COLLEGES USE THE TARIFF?

The Tariff provides a facility to help universities and colleges when expressing entrance requirements and when making conditional offers. Entry requirements and conditional offers expressed as Tariff points will often require a minimum level of achievement in a specified subject (for example '300 points to include grade A at A level chemistry', or '260 points including SQA Higher grade B in mathematics').

Use of the Tariff may also vary from department to department at any one institution, and may in some cases be dependent on the programme being offered.

WHAT QUALIFICATIONS ARE INCLUDED IN THE TARIFF?

The following qualifications are included in the UCAS Tariff. See the number on the qualification title to find the relevant section of the Tariff table.

1   AAT NVQ level 3 in Accounting
2   Advanced Diploma
3   Advanced Extension Awards
4   Advanced Placement Programme
5   Asset Languages Advanced Stage (from 2010 entry onwards)
6   British Horse Society Stage 3 Horse Knowledge & Care, Stage 3 Riding and Preliminary Teacher's Certificate
7   BTEC Early Years
8   BTEC National Award, National Certificate and National Diploma
9   CACHE Diploma in Child Care and Education
10   Cambridge Pre-U
11   Certificate of Personal Effectiveness (COPE)
12   Diploma in Fashion Retail
13   Diploma in Foundation Studies (Art & Design; Art, Design & Media)
14   EDI Level 3 Certificate in Accounting, Certificate in Accounting (IAS)
15   Extended Project
16   Free-standing Mathematics qualifications
17   GCE AS, AS Double Award, A level, A level Double Award and A level with additional AS
18   Higher Sports Leader Award
19   Institute of Financial Services, Certificate and Diploma in Financial Studies
20   International Baccalaureate Diploma
21   International Baccalaureate Certificate
22   iMedia Users (iMedia) Certificate and Diploma
23   IT for Professionals (iPRO) Certificate and Diploma
24   Irish Leaving Certificate - Higher and Ordinary levels
25   Key Skills at levels 2, 3 and 4
26   Music examinations at grades 6, 7 and 8
27   OCR National Certificate, National Diploma and National Extended Diploma
28   Progression Diploma (from 2010 entry onwards)
29   Scottish Higher and Advanced Higher, Skills for Work Higher, and National Progression Awards
30   Speech and Drama examinations at grades 6, 7 and 8 Performance Studies
31   Welsh Baccalaureate Advanced Diploma

Updates on the Tariff, including details on the incorporation of any new qualifications, are posted on **www.ucas.com.**

UCAS TARIFF TABLES

1

AAT NVQ LEVEL 3 IN ACCOUNTING	
GRADE	TARIFF POINTS
PASS	160

2

ADVANCED DIPLOMA

Advanced Diploma = Progression Diploma plus Additional & Specialist Learning (ASL). Please see the appropriate qualification to calculate the ASL score. ASL has a maximum Tariff score of 140. Please see the Progression Diploma (Table 28) for Tariff scores

3

ADVANCED EXTENSION AWARDS	
GRADE	TARIFF POINTS
DISTINCTION	40
MERIT	20

Points for Advanced Extension Awards are over and above those gained form the A level grade

4

ADVANCED PLACEMENT PROGRAMME (US & CANADA)	
GRADE	TARIFF POINTS
Group A	
5	120
4	90
3	60
Group B	
5	50
4	35
3	20

5

ASSET LANGUAGES ADVANCED STAGE			
GRADE	TARIFF POINTS	GRADE	TARIFF POINTS
Speaking		Listening	
GRADE 12	28	GRADE 12	25
GRADE 11	20	GRADE 11	18
GRADE 10	12	GRADE 10	11
Reading		Writing	
GRADE 12	25	GRADE 12	25
GRADE 11	18	GRADE 11	18
GRADE 10	11	GRADE 10	11

Points for Asset Languages come into effect for entry into higher education from 2010 onwards

6

BRITISH HORSE SOCIETY	
GRADE	TARIFF POINTS
Stage 3 Horse Knowledge & Care	
PASS	35
Stage 3 Riding	
PASS	35
Preliminary Teacher's Certificate	
PASS	35

Awarded by Equestrian Qualifications (GB) Ltd (EQL) on behalf of British Horse Society

7

BTEC EARLY YEARS					
GRADE	TARIFF POINTS	GRADE	TARIFF POINTS	GRADE	TARIFF POINTS
Theory				Practical	
Diploma		Certificate			
DDD	320	DD	200	D	120
DDM	280	DM	160	M	80
DMM	240	MM	120	P	40
MMM	220	MP	80		
MMP	160	PP	40		
MPP	120				
PPP	80				

8

BTEC NATIONALS					
GRADE	TARIFF POINTS	GRADE	TARIFF POINTS	GRADE	TARIFF POINTS
National Diploma		National Certificate		National Award	
DDD	360	DD	240	D	120
DDM	320	DM	200	M	80
DMM	280	MM	160	P	40
MMM	240	MP	120		
MMP	200	PP	80		
MPP	160				
PPP	120				

9

CACHE DIPLOMA IN CHILD CARE & EDUCATION			
GRADE	TARIFF POINTS	GRADE	TARIFF POINTS
Theory		Practical	
AA	240	A	120
BB	200	B	100
CC	160	C	80
DD	120	D	60
EE	80	E	40

10

CAMBRIDGE PRE-U					
GRADE	TARIFF POINTS	GRADE	TARIFF POINTS	GRADE	TARIFF POINTS
Principal Subject		Global Perspectives and Research		Short Course	
D1	TBC	D1	TBC	D1	TBC
D2	145	D2	140	D2	TBC
D3	130	D3	126	D3	60
M1	115	M1	112	M1	53
M2	101	M2	98	M2	46
M3	87	M3	84	M3	39
P1	73	P1	70	P1	32
P2	59	P2	56	P2	26
P3	46	P3	42	P3	20

Points for PRE-U come into effect for entry into higher education from 2010 onwards

11

CERTIFICATE OF PERSONAL EFFECTIVENESS (COPE)	
GRADE	TARIFF POINTS
PASS	70

Points are awarded for the Certificate of Personal Effectiveness (COPE) awarded by ASDAN and CCEA

12

DIPLOMA IN FASHION RETAIL	
GRADE	TARIFF POINTS
DISTINCTION	160
MERIT	120
PASS	80

Awarded by ABC Awards

13

DIPLOMA IN FOUNDATION STUDIES (ART & DESIGN, AND ART, DESIGN & MEDIA)	
GRADE	TARIFF POINTS
DISTINCTION	285
MERIT	225
PASS	165

Points are awarded for Edexcel Level 3 BTEC Diploma in Foundation Studies (Art & Design) and Level 3 Diploma in Foundation Studies (Art, Design & Media) awarded by ABC Awards and WJEC

14

EDI LEVEL 3 CERTIFICATE IN ACCOUNTING AND CERTIFICATE IN ACCOUNTING (IAS)	
GRADE	TARIFF POINTS
DISTINCTION	120
MERIT	90
PASS	70

15

EXTENDED PROJECT (STAND ALONE)	
GRADE	TARIFF POINTS
A*	70
A	60
B	50
C	40
D	30
E	20

Points for the Extended Project cannot be counted if taken as part of Progression/Advanced Diploma

16

FREE-STANDING MATHEMATICS	
GRADE	TARIFF POINTS
A	20
B	17
C	13
D	10
E	7

Covers free-standing Mathematics - Additional Maths, Using and Applying Statistics, Working with Algebraic and Graphical Techniques, Modelling with Calculus

UCAS TARIFF TABLES

17

	GCE								
GRADE	TARIFF POINTS	GRADE	TARIFF POINTS	GRADE	TARIFF POINTS	GRADE	TARIFF POINTS	GRADE	TARIFF POINTS
GCE Double Award		A level with additional AS (9 units)		GCE A level		GCE AS		GCE AS Double Award	
A*A*	280	A*A	200	A*	140	A	60	AA	120
A*A	260	AA	180	A	120	B	50	AB	110
AA	240	AB	170	B	100	C	40	BB	100
AB	220	BB	150	C	80	D	30	BC	90
BB	200	BC	140	D	60	E	20	CC	80
BC	180	CC	120	E	40			CD	70
CC	160	CD	110					DD	60
CD	140	DD	90					DE	50
DD	120	DE	80					EE	40
DE	100	EE	60						
EE	80								

18

HIGHER SPORTS LEADER AWARD	
GRADE	TARIFF POINTS
PASS	30

19

INSTITUTE OF FINANCIAL SERVICES			
GRADE	TARIFF POINTS	GRADE	TARIFF POINTS
Certificate in Financial Studies (CeFS)		Diploma in Financial Studies (DipFS)	
A	60	A	60
B	50	B	50
C	40	C	40
D	30	D	30
E	20	E	20

Completion of both qualifications will result in a maximum of 120 UCAS Tariff points

20

INTERNATIONAL BACCALAUREATE (IB) DIPLOMA				INTERNATIONAL BACCALAUREATE (IB) DIPLOMA (REVISED FOR 2010 ENTRY ONWARDS)			
GRADE	TARIFF POINTS	GRADE	TARIFF POINTS	GRADE	TARIFF POINTS	GRADE	TARIFF POINTS
45	768	34	512	45	720	34	479
44	744	33	489	44	698	33	457
43	722	32	466	43	676	32	435
42	698	31	422	42	654	31	413
41	675	30	419	41	632	30	392
40	652	29	396	40	611	29	370
39	628	28	373	39	589	28	348
38	605	27	350	38	567	27	326
37	582	26	326	37	545	26	304
36	559	25	303	36	523	25	282
35	535	24	280	35	501	24	260

UCAS TARIFF TABLES

21

INTERNATIONAL BACCALAUREATE (IB) CERTIFICATE					
GRADE	TARIFF POINTS	GRADE	TARIFF POINTS	GRADE	TARIFF POINTS
Higher Level		Standard Level		Core	
7	130	7	70	3	120
6	110	6	59	2	80
5	80	5	43	1	40
4	50	4	27	0	10
3	20	3	11		

Points for the IB Certificate come into effect for entry into higher education from 2010 onwards

22

iMEDIA USERS (iMEDIA)	
GRADE	TARIFF POINTS
DIPLOMA	66
CERTIFICATE	40

Awarded by OCR

23

IT PROFESSIONALS (iPRO)	
GRADE	TARIFF POINTS
DIPLOMA	100
CERTIFICATE	80

Awarded by OCR

24

IRISH LEAVING CERTIFICATE			
GRADE	TARIFF POINTS	GRADE	TARIFF POINTS
Higher		Ordinary	
A1	90	A1	39
A2	77	A2	26
B1	71	B1	20
B2	64	B2	14
B3	58	B3	7
C1	52		
C2	45		
C3	39		
D1	33		
D2	26		
D3	20		

25

KEY SKILLS	
GRADE	TARIFF POINTS
LEVEL 4	30
LEVEL 3	20
LEVEL 2	10

26

MUSIC EXAMINATIONS					
GRADE	TARIFF POINTS	GRADE	TARIFF POINTS	GRADE	TARIFF POINTS
Practical					
Grade 8		Grade 7		Grade 6	
DISTINCTION	75	DISTINCTION	60	DISTINCTION	45
MERIT	70	MERIT	55	MERIT	40
PASS	55	PASS	40	PASS	25
Theory					
Grade 8		Grade 7		Grade 6	
DISTINCTION	30	DISTINCTION	20	DISTINCTION	15
MERIT	25	MERIT	15	MERIT	10
PASS	20	PASS	10	PASS	5

Points shown are for the ABRSM, Guildhall, LCMM, Rockschool and Trinity College London Advanced level music examinations

UCAS TARIFF TABLES

27

OCR NATIONALS							
GRADE	TARIFF POINTS	GRADE	TARIFF POINTS	GRADE	TARIFF POINTS		
National Extended Diploma		National Diploma		National Certificate			
D1	360	D	240	D	120		
D2/M1	320	M1	200	M	80		
M2	280	M2/P1	160	P	40		
M3	240	P2	120				
P1	200	P3	80				
P2	160						
P3	120						

28

PROGRESSION DIPLOMA	
GRADE	TARIFF POINTS
A*	350
A	300
B	250
C	200
D	150
E	100

Points for the Progression Diploma come into effect for entry to higher education from 2010 onwards.

Advanced Diploma = Progression Diploma plus Additional & Specialist Learning (ASL). Please see the appropriate qualification to calculate the ASL score. ASL has a maximum Tariff score of 140

29

SCOTTISH QUALIFICATIONS				SCOTTISH QUALIFICATIONS (REVISED FOR 2010 ENTRY ONWARDS)			
GRADE	TARIFF POINTS	GRADE	TARIFF POINTS	GRADE	TARIFF POINTS	GRADE	TARIFF POINTS
Advanced Higher		Higher		Advanced Higher		Higher	
A	120	A	72	A	130	A	80
B	100	B	60	B	110	B	65
C	80	C	48	C	90	C	50
D	72	D	42	D	72	D	36
				Ungraded Higher		NPA PC Passport	
				PASS	45	PASS	45

30

SPEECH & DRAMA EXAMINATIONS							
GRADE	TARIFF POINTS	GRADE	TARIFF POINTS	GRADE	TARIFF POINTS	GRADE	TARIFF POINTS
PCertLAM**		Grade 8		Grade 7		Grade 6	
DISTINCTION	90	DISTINCTION	65	DISTINCTION	55	DISTINCTION	40
MERIT	80	MERIT	60	MERIT	50	MERIT	35
PASS	60	PASS	45	PASS	35	PASS	20

Points shown are for ESB, LAMDA, LCMM and Trinity Guildhall Advanced level speech and drama examinations accredited in the National Qualifications Framework. A full list of the subjects covered is available on the UCAS website.

31

WELSH BACCALAUREATE CORE	
GRADE	TARIFF POINTS
PASS	120

These points are for the Core and are awarded only when a candidate achieves the Welsh Baccalaureate Advanced Diploma

Results

4

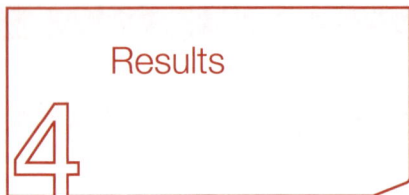

Step 4 – Results

We receive many exam results direct from the exam boards – check the list at **www.ucas.com**. If your qualification is listed, you don't need to send your results to us or the universities and colleges. Check Track at **www.ucas.com** to see if you've got a place on your chosen course.

If your qualification is listed, we send your results to the universities and colleges that you have accepted as your firm and insurance choices. If your qualification is not listed, you must send your exam results to the universities and colleges where you are holding offers.

You should arrange your holidays so that you are at home when your exam results are published because, if there are any issues to discuss, admissions tutors will want to speak to you in person.

After you have received your exam results check Track to find out if you have a place on your chosen course.

If you have met all the conditions for your firm choice, the university or college will confirm that you have a place. Sometimes, they may still confirm you have a place even if you have not quite met all the offer conditions; or they may offer you a place on a similar course.

If you have not met the conditions of your firm choice and the university or college has not confirmed your place, but you have met all the conditions of your insurance offer, the university or college will confirm that you have a place.

When a university or college tells us that you have a place, we send you confirmation by letter.

WHAT IF YOU DON'T HAVE A PLACE?

If you have not met the conditions of either your firm or insurance choice, and your chosen universities or colleges have not confirmed your place, you are eligible for Clearing. In Clearing you can apply for courses that still have vacancies. Clearing operates from mid-July to late September 2010 (page 102).

BETTER RESULTS THAN EXPECTED?

If you obtain exam results that meet and exceed the conditions of the offer for your firm choice, you can for a short period look for an alternative place, whilst still keeping your original firm choice (page 103).

> Next steps

5

Step 5 – Next steps

IF YOU FIND YOURSELF IN CLEARING, YOU WILL NEED TO

Find a course you like – do your research thoroughly and quickly. You could consider related or alternative subjects or perhaps apply for the subject you want in combination with another. Your teachers or careers advisers or the universities and colleges themselves can provide useful guidance. If your results are reasonable, and you are flexible about where and what you want to study, you have every chance of finding a place on a suitable course.

Talk to the institutions – don't be afraid to call them. Prepare a list of what you will say to them about:

- why you want to study the course
- why you want to study at their institution
- what relevant employment or activities you have done that relate to the course
- your grades

and have ready your:

- Personal ID
- Clearing number.

Getting an offer – don't be pressured into doing something you don't like but once you find a course you will enjoy, stick with it.

IF YOUR RESULTS MEET AND EXCEED YOUR CONDITIONAL FIRM OFFER, YOU CAN ADJUST YOUR PLACE

You may decide to research alternative institutions and courses. Talk to your school or college adviser first. If you find a course that you think you may be qualified for and which has places available, you need to talk to the new institution to adjust your place.

There are no published vacancies in Adjustment so you'll need to talk to the institutions – have all your information ready before you call:

- full details of your exam results
- why you want to change your course
- why you want to study at their institution
- what relevant employment or activities you have done that relate to the course
- your Personal ID.

You may be able to adjust to a deferred entry place if there are no places left and if your results meet the course entry requirements – you do not need to withdraw and reapply. Be aware that you have only five calendar days (including weekends) to consider changing your course in these circumstances – you must complete both your research and your negotiation within this time.

IF YOU ARE STILL WITHOUT A PLACE TO STUDY:

You could re-sit your exams and try again next year, find employment, decide to do a further education course or apply for a part-time course and a part-time job. Seek advice from your school or college or careers office.

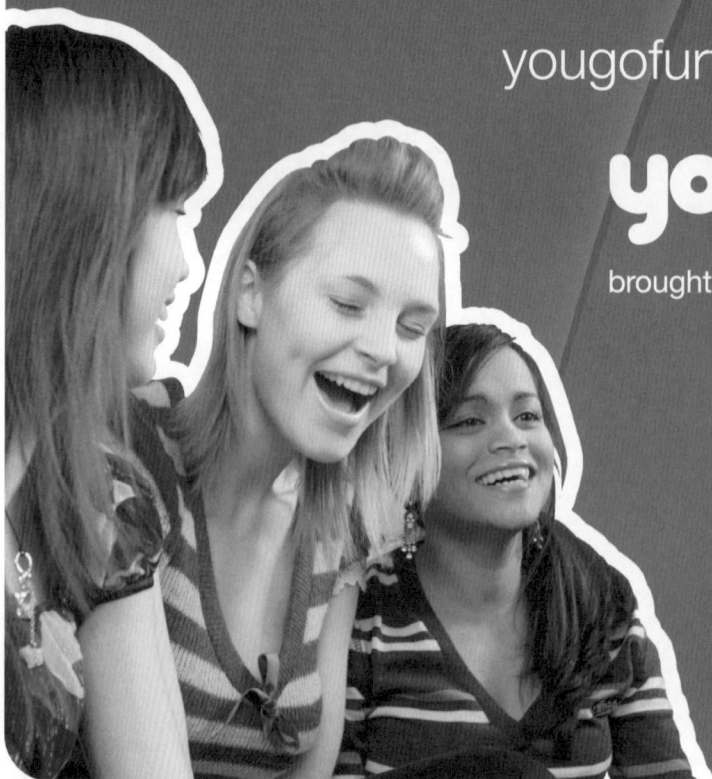

6

Starting university
or college

Step 6 – Starting university or college

Make sure you have everything ready, such as accommodation, finances, travel arrangements, books and equipment required for the course.

Congratulations! Now you have your place at university or college you will need to make plans on how to get there, where to live and how to finance it.

Where to live - Unless you are planning to live at home, your university or college will usually provide you with guidance on how to find somewhere to live. The earlier you contact them the better your chance of finding a suitable range of options to choose from.

Student finance – You will need to budget for living costs, accommodation, travel, books and tuition fees. Tuition fees vary depending on the course and university you choose, and are shown on Course Search at **www.ucas.com**. Help is available from some universities and colleges in the form of bursaries and scholarships. Details of these bursaries and scholarships can also be found on Course Search.

Yougofurther.co.uk – You might have already registered for **www.yougofurther.co.uk**, the social community website brought to you by UCAS that is exclusively for students. The site allows you to make friends with other applicants who are going to the same university or college and/or who are going to be on the same course, or who live in your area. It has all the essential information you need for life at university. Whether it's jobs, money, travel, housing or healthy living – yougo's got it covered.

Useful contacts

For information relating to the UCAS application process, please contact the UCAS Customer Service Unit on 0871 468 0 468. Calls from BT landlines within the UK will cost no more than 9p per minute. The cost of calls from mobiles and other networks may vary.

If you have hearing difficulties, you can call the RNID typetalk service on 18001 0871 468 0 468 (outside the UK +44 151 494 1260). Calls are charged at normal rates.

CAREERS ADVICE

Connexions is for you if you live in England, are aged 13 to 19 and want advice on getting to where you want to be in life.

Connexions personal advisers can give you information, advice and practical help with all sorts of things, like choosing subjects at school or mapping out your future career options. They can help you with anything that might be affecting you at school, college, work or in your personal or family life.

For where to find your local office, look at **www.connexions.gov.uk**.

Careers Scotland provides a starting point for anyone looking for careers information, advice or guidance. **www.careers-scotland.org.uk**.

Careers Wales – Wales' national all-age careers guidance service.
www.careerswales.com.

Northern Ireland Careers Service website for the new, all-age careers guidance service in Northern Ireland.
www.careersserviceni.com.

Learndirect – Not sure what job you want? Need help to decide which course to do? Give learndirect a call on 0800 101 901 or, for Scotland, 0808 100 9000. **www.learndirect.co.uk.**
www.learndirectscotland.com.

YEAR OUT

For useful information on taking a year out, see **www.gap-year.com**.

The Year Out Group website is packed with information and guidance for young people and their parents and advisers.
www.yearoutgroup.org.

STUDENT SUPPORT

Each country in the UK has its own rules and procedures, and you should check the websites for the country where you normally live for more information. The following websites should give you information about what grants and loans you may be eligible to apply for and how you can apply.

If your family lives in England, you should visit, **www.direct.gov.uk/studentfinance**

If your family lives in Wales, you should visit **www.studentfinancewales.co.uk** or **www.cyllidmyfyrwyrcymru.co.uk.**

If your family lives in Scotland, you should visit **www.saas.gov.uk.**

If your family lives in Northern Ireland, you should visit **www.studentfinanceni.co.uk**

If your family lives in Guernsey, Jersey or the Isle of Man, you should visit **www.gov.gg/, www.gov.je/** or **www.gov.im/.**

Disabled Students' Allowance
If you have a disability or specific learning difficulty, you may be able to apply for a Disabled Students' Allowance. To find out more you should visit the websites listed above and search on Disabled Student.

Essential reading

UCAS has brought together the best books and resources you need to make the important decisions regarding entry to higher education. With guidance on choosing courses, finding the right institution, information about student finance, admissions tests, gap years and lots more, you can find the most trusted guides at www.ucasbooks.com.

The publications listed on the following pages are available through www.ucasbooks.com or from UCAS Publication Services unless otherwise stated. Postage and packing charges are not included in the price. You will be advised of the postage and packing charge when placing your order.

UCAS Publication Services

UCAS Publication Services
PO Box 130
Cheltenham
Gloucestershire GL52 3ZF

f: 01242 544 806
e: publicationservices@ucas.ac.uk
// www.ucas.com
// www.ucasbooks.com

NEED HELP COMPLETING YOUR APPLICATION?

How to Complete your UCAS Application 2010

A must for anyone applying through UCAS. Contains advice on the preparation needed, a step-by-step guide to filling out the UCAS application, information on the UCAS process and useful tips for completing the personal statement.

Published by Trotman

Price £12.99

Insider's Guide to Applying to University

Full of honest insights, this is a thorough guide to the application process. It reveals advice from careers advisers and current students, guidance on making sense of university information and choosing courses. Also includes tips for the personal statement, interviews, admissions tests, UCAS Extra and Clearing.

Published by Trotman

Price £12.99

How to Write a Winning UCAS Personal Statement

The personal statement is your chance to stand out from the crowd. Based on information from admissions tutors, this book will help you sell yourself. It includes specific guidance for over 30 popular subjects, common mistakes to avoid, information on what admissions tutors look for, and much more.

Published by Trotman

Price £12.99

CHOOSING COURSES

Progression Series 2010 entry

UCAS, in conjunction with GTI Specialist Publishers, has produced a series of ten titles for 2010 entry. The 'Progression to…' titles are designed to help you access good quality, useful information on some of the most competitive subject areas. The books cover advice on applying through UCAS, routes to qualifications, course details, job prospects, case studies and career advice.

Progression to…

Art and Design

Economics, Finance and Accountancy

Engineering and Mathematics

Health and Social Care

Law

Media and Performing Arts

Medicine, Dentistry and Optometry

Psychology

Sports Science and Physiotherapy

Teaching and Education

Published by UCAS

Price £15.99 each

UCAS Parent Guide

Free of charge.

Order online at **www.ucas.com/parents**

or call 0845 468 0 468.

Open Days 2009

Attending open days, taster courses and higher education conventions is an important part of the application process. This publication makes planning attendance at these events quick and easy.

Published annually by UCAS in association with Cambridge Occupational Analysts.

Price £3.50

Getting in, Getting on 2010

Conventions have become a central part of the post-16 careers education and guidance programme. This publication has been designed to be used before, during and after the event. It can make a difference.
Published by UCAS
Price £16

'Getting into…' guides

Clear and concise guides to help applicants secure places. They include qualifications required, advice on applying, tests, interviews and case studies. The guides give an honest view and discuss current issues and careers.

Getting into Business and Management Courses
Getting into Oxford and Cambridge
Getting into US and Canadian Universities
Getting into Veterinary School
Published by Trotman
Price £12.99 each

Choosing Your Degree Course & University

With so many universities and courses to choose from, it is not an easy decision for students embarking on their journey to higher education. This guide will offer expert guidance on the questions students need to ask when considering the opportunities available.
Published by Trotman 11th Edition
Price £22.99

Degree Course Descriptions

Providing details of the nature of degree courses, the descriptions in this book are written by heads of departments and senior lecturers at major universities. Each description contains an overview of the course area, details of course structures, career opportunities and more.
Published by COA
Price £12.99

Insider's Guide to Applying to University

Full of honest insights, this is a thorough guide to the application process. It reveals advice from careers advisers and current students, guidance on making sense of university information and choosing courses. Also includes tips for the personal statement, interviews, admissions tests, UCAS Extra and Clearing.
Published by Trotman
Price £12.99

CHOOSING WHERE TO STUDY

The Virgin 2010 Guide to British Universities

An insider's guide to choosing a university or college. Written by students and using independent statistics, this guide evaluates what you get from a higher education institution.
Published by Virgin
Price £15.99

Times Good University Guide 2010

How do you find the best university for the subject you wish to study? You need a guide that evaluates the quality of what is available, giving facts, figures and comparative assessments of universities. The rankings provide hard data, analysed, interpreted and presented by a team of experts.
Published by The Times
Price £15.99

Guardian University Guide 2010

Packed with no-nonsense advice, this book takes prospective students through every process they will encounter: from applications to interviews, accommodation to finances. The Guardian subject ratings are based on the UCAS entry Tariffs so that students can judge for themselves which are the best universities available to them.
Published by The Guardian
Price £15.99

The Daily Telegraph Guide to UK Universities 2010

Includes profiles of all institutions offering higher education courses, with information from current students providing a unique, independent insight into what each institution is really like. Included are details of the location, housing, cost of living, sports, nightlife, information on fees and bursaries and more.

Published by Trotman

Price £17.99

Getting into the UK's Best Universities and Courses

This book is for those who set their goals high and dream of studying on a highly regarded course at a good university. It provides information on selecting the best courses for a subject, the application and personal statement, interviews, results day, timescales for applications and much more.

Published by Trotman

Price £12.99

FINANCIAL INFORMATION

Students' Money Matters 2010

With graduate debt increasing, this guide provides invaluable information for students about loans, overdrafts, work experience, jobs and accommodation. Also includes advice on budgeting, borrowing and top-up fees.

Published by Trotman

Price £16.99

University Scholarships, Awards & Bursaries

Students embarking on HE courses face an increasingly challenging financial situation. This book enables applicants and current students to find the support that may help them make ends meet. Packed with information on virtually all awards available.

Published by Trotman 7th Edition

Price £22.99

CAREERS PLANNING

What Do Graduates Do?

A comprehensive look at graduate employment. Providing data detailing the first destinations of first-degree and HND graduates, this guide profiles how many leavers enter employment or further study and how many are unemployed. To complement the data, there are articles and editorial for each subject area.

Published by Graduate Prospects

Price £14.95

The Careers Directory

An indispensable resource for anyone seeking careers information, covering over 350 careers. It presents up-to-date information in an innovative double-page format. Ideal for students in years 10 to 13 who are considering their futures and for other careers professionals.

Published by COA

Price £15.99

DEFERRING ENTRY

Your Gap Year

The essential book for all young people planning a gap year before continuing with their education. This up-to-date guide provides essential information on specialist gap year programes, as well as the vast range of jobs and voluntary opportunities available to young people around the world.
Published by Crimson Publishing
Price £12.99

Summer Jobs Worldwide 2009

This unique and specialist guide contains over 40,000 jobs for all ages. No other book includes such a variety and wealth of summer work opportunities in Britain and aboard. Anything from horse trainer in Iceland, to a guide for nature walks in Peru, to a yoga centre helper in Greece, to an animal keeper for London Zoo, can be found.
Published by Crimson Publishing
Price £12.99

Teaching English Abroad

The definitive and acclaimed guide to opportunities for trained and untrained teachers across the world. With the field of teaching English as a foreign language booming, this guide offers extensive information for anyone wishing to teach English abroad. Including listings of recruitment organisations, a directory of more than 380 courses, and 1,150 language school addresses to contact for jobs.
Published by Crimson Publishing
Price £14.99

Please note all publications incur a postage and packing charge. All information was correct at the time of printing.

For a full list of publications, please visit
www.ucasbooks.com.

Confused about courses?
Indecisive about institutions?
Stressed about student life?
Unsure about UCAS?
Frowning over finance?

Help is available.

Visit www.ucasbooks.com to view our range
of over 75 books covering all aspects
of entry into higher education.

www.ucasbooks.com

Courses

Courses

Keen to get started on your sports science and physiotherapy career? This section contains details of the various degree courses available at UK institutions.

EXPLAINING THE LIST OF COURSES

We list the universities and colleges by their UCAS institution codes. Within each institution, courses are listed first by award type (such as BA, BSc, FdA, HND, MA and many others), then alphabetically by course title.

You might find some courses showing an award type '(Mod)', which indicates a combined degree that might be modular in design. A small number of courses have award type '(FYr)'. This indicates a 12-month foundation course, after which students can choose to apply for a degree course. In either case, you should contact the university or college for further details.

Generally speaking, when a course comprises two or more subjects, the word used to connect the subjects indicates the make-up of the award: 'Subject A and Subject B' is a joint award, where both subjects carry equal weight; 'Subject A with Subject B' is a major/minor award, where Subject A accounts for at least 60% of your study. If the title shows 'Subject A/Subject B', it may indicate that students can decide on the weighting of the subjects at the end of the first year. You should check with the university or college for full details.

Each entry in the UCAS sections shows the UCAS course code and the duration of the course. Where known, the entry contains details of the minimum qualification requirements for the course, as supplied to UCAS by the universities and colleges. Bear in mind that possessing the minimum qualifications does not guarantee acceptance to the course: there may be far more applicants than places. You may be asked to attend an interview, present a portfolio or sit an admissions test.

Before applying for any course, you are advised to contact the university or college to check any changes in entry requirements and to see if any new courses have come on stream since the lists were approved for publication. To make this easy, each institution's entry starts with their address, email, phone and fax details, as well as their website address. You will also find it useful to check the Entry Profiles section of Course Search at **www.ucas.com**.

> **Unlock your potential**
It's as easy as 1, 2, 3.

1 **Search**

Use Course Search to look for courses in your subject;
find out about your chosen universities and colleges
and lots more.

2 **Apply**

Use our online system Apply to make your application to
higher education.

3 **Track**

Then use Track to monitor the progress of your application.

UCAS   helping students into higher education   **www.ucas.com**

SPORTS SCIENCE

A40 ABERYSTWYTH UNIVERSITY

WELCOME CENTRE, ABERYSTWYTH UNIVERSITY
PENGLAIS CAMPUS
ABERYSTWYTH
CEREDIGION SY23 3FB
t: 01970 622021 f: 01970 627410
e: ug-admissions@aber.ac.uk
// www.aber.ac.uk

CD64 BSc Equine and Human Sport Science
Duration: 3FT Hon

Entry Requirements: *GCE:* 240. *IB:* 26.

A60 ANGLIA RUSKIN UNIVERSITY

BISHOP HALL LANE
CHELMSFORD
ESSEX CM1 1SQ
t: 0845 271 3333 f: 01245 251789
e: answers@anglia.ac.uk
// www.anglia.ac.uk

C602 BSc Coaching Science
Duration: 3FT Hon

Entry Requirements: *GCE:* 180. *SQAH:* CCCC. *SQAAH:* CC. *IB:* 24.

C600 BSc Sports Science
Duration: 3FT Hon

Entry Requirements: *GCE:* 180. *SQAH:* BCCC. *SQAAH:* CC. *IB:* 24.

B06 BANGOR UNIVERSITY

BANGOR
GWYNEDD LL57 2DG
t: 01248 382016/2017 f: 01248 370451
e: admissions@bangor.ac.uk
// www.bangor.ac.uk

QC36 BA English Language and Sports Science
Duration: 3FT Hon

Entry Requirements: *GCE:* 260-280. *IB:* 28.

CL65 BA Health & Social Care/Sports Science
Duration: 3FT Hon

Entry Requirements: *GCE:* 260-280. *IB:* 28.

CR61 BA Sports Science/French (4 years)
Duration: 4FT Hon

Entry Requirements: *GCE:* 260-280. *IB:* 28.

CL63 BA Sports Science/Sociology
Duration: 3FT Hon

Entry Requirements: *GCE:* 260-280. *IB:* 28.

XCJ6 BSc Astudiaethau Plentyndod/Gwyddor Chwaraeon
Duration: 3FT Hon

Entry Requirements: *GCE:* 260-280. *IB:* 28.

C602 BSc Sport Science (Outdoor Activities)
Duration: 3FT Hon

Entry Requirements: *GCE:* 260-280. *IB:* 28.

C6CV BSc Sport Science with Psychology
Duration: 3FT Hon

Entry Requirements: *GCE:* 260-280. *IB:* 28.

CQ6M BSc Sport Science/Cymraeg
Duration: 3FT Hon

Entry Requirements: *GCE:* 260-280. *IB:* 28.

CQ6C BSc Sport Science/Linguistics
Duration: 3FT Hon

Entry Requirements: *GCE:* 260-280. *IB:* 28.

CL6K BSc Sport Science/Social Policy
Duration: 3FT Hon

Entry Requirements: *GCE:* 260-280. *IB:* 28.

CR6L BSc Sport Science/Spanish
Duration: 4FT Hon

Entry Requirements: *GCE:* 260-280. *IB:* 28.

C600 BSc Sports Science
Duration: 3FT Hon

Entry Requirements: *GCE:* 260-280. *IB:* 28.

B15 BASINGSTOKE COLLEGE OF TECHNOLOGY

WORTING ROAD
BASINGSTOKE RG21 8TN
t: (Main) 01256 354141 f: 01256 306444
e: info@bcot.ac.uk
// www.bcot.ac.uk

006C HND Sport and Exercise Sciences
Duration: 2FT HND

Entry Requirements: *GCE:* 120. *BTEC NC:* PP. *BTEC ND:* PPP.

B22 UNIVERSITY OF BEDFORDSHIRE
PARK SQUARE
LUTON
BEDS LU1 3JU
t: 01582 489286 f: 01582 489323
e: admissions@beds.ac.uk
// www.beds.ac.uk

C603 BSc Applied Sport Science (Level 3 only)
Duration: 1FT Hon

Entry Requirements: HND required.

C600 BSc Sport and Exercise Science
Duration: 3FT Hon

Entry Requirements: Contact the institution for details.

C613 BSc Sports Science and Personal Training
Duration: 3FT Hon

Entry Requirements: Contact the institution for details.

B32 THE UNIVERSITY OF BIRMINGHAM
EDGBASTON
BIRMINGHAM B15 2TT
t: 0121 415 8900 f: 0121 414 7159
e: admissions@bham.ac.uk
// www.bham.ac.uk

CF62 BSc Sports Science and Materials Technology
Duration: 3FT Hon

Entry Requirements: GCE: BBB. SQAH: BBBBB. SQAAH: BBB. IB: 30.

B44 THE UNIVERSITY OF BOLTON
DEANE ROAD
BOLTON BL3 5AB
t: 01204 900600 f: 01204 399074
e: enquiries@bolton.ac.uk
// www.bolton.ac.uk

C603 BSc Sport & Exercise Science
Duration: 3FT Hon

Entry Requirements: GCE: 200. IB: 20. BTEC NC: DM. BTEC ND: MMP.

B60 BRADFORD COLLEGE: AN ASSOCIATE COLLEGE OF LEEDS METROPOLITAN UNIVERSITY
GREAT HORTON ROAD
BRADFORD
WEST YORKSHIRE BD7 1AY
t: 01274 433333 f: 01274 433241
e: admissions@bradfordcollege.ac.uk
// www.bradfordcollege.ac.uk

C600 FdSc Sports Science
Duration: 2FT Hon

Entry Requirements: Contact the institution for details.

B79 BRISTOL FILTON COLLEGE
FILTON AVENUE
BRISTOL BS34 7AT
t: 0117 909 2255 f: 0117 931 2233
e: info@filton.ac.uk
// www.filton.ac.uk

006C HND Sport & Exercise Science
Duration: 2FT HND

Entry Requirements: GCE: 160. BTEC ND: MPP. Interview required.

B80 UNIVERSITY OF THE WEST OF ENGLAND, BRISTOL
FRENCHAY CAMPUS
COLDHARBOUR LANE
BRISTOL BS16 1QY
t: +44 (0)117 32 83333 f: +44 (0)117 32 82810
e: admissions@uwe.ac.uk
// www.uwe.ac.uk

DCK6 FdSc Equine Sports Science
Duration: 2FT Fdg

Entry Requirements: GCE: 100-140.

B84 BRUNEL UNIVERSITY
UXBRIDGE
MIDDLESEX UB8 3PH
t: 01895 265265 f: 01895 269790
e: admissions@brunel.ac.uk
// www.brunel.ac.uk

C6N1 BSc Business Studies and Sport Sciences
Duration: 3FT Hon

Entry Requirements: GCE: 350. IB: 32. BTEC ND: DDD.

B94 BUCKINGHAMSHIRE NEW UNIVERSITY

QUEEN ALEXANDRA ROAD
HIGH WYCOMBE
BUCKS HP11 2JZ

t: 0800 0565 660 f: 01494 605023
e: admissions@bucks.ac.uk

// www.bucks.ac.uk

CX6C BSc Sports Science and Coaching Studies

Duration: 3FT Hon

Entry Requirements: *GCE:* 200-240.

C10 CANTERBURY CHRIST CHURCH UNIVERSITY

NORTH HOLMES ROAD
CANTERBURY
KENT CT1 1QU

t: 01227 782900 f: 01227 782888
e: admissions@canterbury.ac.uk

// www.canterbury.ac.uk

CC16 BSc Biosciences and Sport & Exercise Science

Duration: 3FT Hon

Entry Requirements: *IB:* 24.

C1C6 BSc/BA Biosciences with Sport & Exercise Science

Duration: 3FT Hon

Entry Requirements: *IB:* 24.

C20 UNIVERSITY OF WALES INSTITUTE, CARDIFF

PO BOX 377
LLANDAFF CAMPUS
WESTERN AVENUE
CARDIFF CF5 2SG

t: 029 2041 6070 f: 029 2041 6286
e: admissions@uwic.ac.uk

// www.uwic.ac.uk

C605 BSc Sport & Exercise Science (Intercalated)

Duration: 1FT Hon

Entry Requirements: Interview required.

C55 UNIVERSITY OF CHESTER

PARKGATE ROAD
CHESTER CH1 4BJ

t: 01244 511000 f: 01244 511300
e: enquiries@chester.ac.uk

// www.chester.ac.uk

NC56 BA Marketing and Sport & Exercise Sciences

Duration: 3FT Hon

Entry Requirements: *Foundation:* Pass. *GCE:* 240. *SQAH:* BBBB. *IB:* 24. *BTEC NC:* DM. *BTEC ND:* MMM.

CR62 BA Sport & Exercise Sciences and German

Duration: 4FT Hon

Entry Requirements: *GCE:* 240. *SQAH:* BBBB. *IB:* 24. *BTEC NC:* DM. *BTEC ND:* MMM.

C6C1 BSc Sport & Exercise Sciences with Biology

Duration: 3FT Hon

Entry Requirements: *GCE:* 240. *SQAH:* BBBB. *IB:* 24. *BTEC NC:* DM. *BTEC ND:* MMM.

C78 CORNWALL COLLEGE

POOL
REDRUTH
CORNWALL TR15 3RD

t: 01209 616161 f: 01209 611612
e: he.admissions@cornwall.ac.uk

// www.cornwall.ac.uk

CF67 FdSc Marine Sports Science

Duration: 2FT Fdg

Entry Requirements: *GCE:* 120. *IB:* 24. *BTEC NC:* MP. *BTEC ND:* PPP. Interview required.

CB69 FdSc Sport (Pathways to Health & Fitness and Exercise Science)

Duration: 2FT Fdg

Entry Requirements: Contact the institution for details.

CF68 FdSc Surf Science and Technology

Duration: 2FT Fdg

Entry Requirements: *GCE:* 120. *IB:* 24. *BTEC NC:* MP. *BTEC ND:* PPP. Interview required.

C85 COVENTRY UNIVERSITY

THE STUDENT CENTRE
COVENTRY UNIVERSITY
1 GULSON RD
COVENTRY CV1 2JH

t: 024 7615 2222 **f:** 024 7615 2223
e: studentenquiries@coventry.ac.uk

// www.coventry.ac.uk

C600 BSc Sport and Exercise Science

Duration: 3FT/4SW Hon

Entry Requirements: *GCE:* 240. *BTEC NC:* DD. *BTEC ND:* MMM.

CX61 FdSc Strength and Conditioning Science

Duration: 2FT Fdg

Entry Requirements: *GCE:* 80. *BTEC NC:* PP. *BTEC ND:* PPP.

C99 UNIVERSITY OF CUMBRIA

FUSEHILL STREET
CARLISLE
CUMBRIA CA1 2HH

t: 01228 616234 **f:** 01228 616235

// www.cumbria.ac.uk

C600 BSc Sport and Exercise Science

Duration: 3FT Hon

Entry Requirements: *Foundation:* Distinction. *GCE:* 240. *IB:* 28.
BTEC NC: DD. *BTEC ND:* MMM. *OCR ND:* Distinction.

C609 DipHE Sport and Exercise Science

Duration: 2FT Dip

Entry Requirements: *Foundation:* Pass. *GCE:* 80. *IB:* 24. *BTEC NC:*
PP. *BTEC ND:* PPP.

D39 UNIVERSITY OF DERBY

KEDLESTON ROAD
DERBY DE22 1GB

t: 08701 202330 **f:** 01332 597724
e: askadmissions@derby.ac.uk

// www.derby.ac.uk

KC16 BA Architectural Design and Sport & Exercise Studies

Duration: 3FT Hon

Entry Requirements: *Foundation:* Merit. *GCE:* 180-240. *IB:* 26.
BTEC NC: DM. *BTEC ND:* MMP.

VC3P BA Art & Design History and Sport & Exercise Studies

Duration: 3FT Hon

Entry Requirements: Contact the institution for details.

CN6N BA Sport & Exercise Studies and Marketing

Duration: 3FT Hon

Entry Requirements: *Foundation:* Merit. *GCE:* 180-240. *IB:* 26.
BTEC NC: DM. *BTEC ND:* MMP.

VC36 BA/BSc Art & Design History and Sport & Exercise Science

Duration: 3FT Hon

Entry Requirements: Contact the institution for details.

CT67 BA/BSc Sport & Exercise Science and American Studies

Duration: 3FT Hon

Entry Requirements: *Foundation:* Merit. *GCE:* 180-240. *IB:* 26.
BTEC NC: DM. *BTEC ND:* MMP.

CK61 BA/BSc Sport & Exercise Science and Architectural Design

Duration: 3FT Hon

Entry Requirements: *Foundation:* Merit. *GCE:* 180-240. *IB:* 26.
BTEC NC: DM. *BTEC ND:* MMP.

CWPV BA/BSc Sport & Exercise Science and Creative Writing

Duration: 3FT Hon

Entry Requirements: *Foundation:* Merit. *GCE:* 180-240. *IB:* 26.
BTEC NC: DM. *BTEC ND:* MMP.

CW6M BA/BSc Sport & Exercise Science and Dance & Movement Studies

Duration: 3FT Hon

Entry Requirements: *GCE:* 180-240. *BTEC NC:* DM. *BTEC ND:* MMP.

CQP3 BA/BSc Sport & Exercise Science and English

Duration: 3FT Hon

Entry Requirements: *Foundation:* Merit. *GCE:* 180-240. *IB:* 26.
BTEC NC: DM. *BTEC ND:* MMP.

CNQG BA/BSc Sport & Exercise Science and Enterprise Management

Duration: 3FT Hon

Entry Requirements: *Foundation:* Merit. *GCE:* 180-240. *IB:* 26.
BTEC NC: DM. *BTEC ND:* MMP.

CBP3 BA/BSc Sport & Exercise Science and Healing Arts

Duration: 3FT Hon

Entry Requirements: *Foundation:* Merit. *GCE:* 180-240. *IB:* 26.
BTEC NC: DM. *BTEC ND:* MMP.

CN6P BA/BSc Sport & Exercise Science and Human Resources Management
Duration: 3FT Hon

Entry Requirements: *Foundation:* Merit. *GCE:* 180-240. *IB:* 26. *BTEC NC:* DM. *BTEC ND:* MMP.

CM6C BA/BSc Sport & Exercise Science and Law
Duration: 3FT Hon

Entry Requirements: *Foundation:* Merit. *GCE:* 180-240. *IB:* 26. *BTEC NC:* DM. *BTEC ND:* MMP.

CN6M BA/BSc Sport & Exercise Science and Marketing
Duration: 3FT Hon

Entry Requirements: *Foundation:* Merit. *GCE:* 180-240. *IB:* 26. *BTEC NC:* DM. *BTEC ND:* MMP.

CWQ8 BA/BSc Sport & Exercise Science and Media Writing
Duration: 3FT Hon

Entry Requirements: *Foundation:* Merit. *GCE:* 180-240. *IB:* 26. *BTEC NC:* DM. *BTEC ND:* MMP.

CW63 BA/BSc Sport & Exercise Science and Popular Music Production
Duration: 3FT Hon

Entry Requirements: *Foundation:* Merit. *GCE:* 180-240. *IB:* 26. *BTEC NC:* DM. *BTEC ND:* MMP.

C612 BA/BSc Sports Development and Physical Activity & Health
Duration: 3FT Hon

Entry Requirements: Contact the institution for details.

NC86 BA/BSc Travel & Tourism and Sport & Exercise Science
Duration: 3FT Hon

Entry Requirements: *Foundation:* Merit. *GCE:* 180-240. *IB:* 26. *BTEC NC:* DM. *BTEC ND:* MMP.

GCK6 BSc Computer Networks and Sport & Exercise Science
Duration: 3FT Hon

Entry Requirements: Contact the institution for details.

GCL6 BSc Computing and Sport & Exercise Science
Duration: 3FT Hon

Entry Requirements: Contact the institution for details.

CC6C BSc Sport & Exercise Science and Biology
Duration: 3FT Hon

Entry Requirements: *Foundation:* Merit. *GCE:* 180-240. *IB:* 26. *BTEC NC:* DM. *BTEC ND:* MMP.

CG6K BSc Sport & Exercise Science and Computer Networks
Duration: 3FT Hon

Entry Requirements: *Foundation:* Merit. *GCE:* 180-240. *IB:* 26. *BTEC NC:* DM. *BTEC ND:* MMP.

CGP4 BSc Sport & Exercise Science and Computing Management
Duration: 3FT Hon

Entry Requirements: *Foundation:* Merit. *GCE:* 180-240. *IB:* 26. *BTEC NC:* DM. *BTEC ND:* MMP.

CM69 BSc Sport & Exercise Science and Criminology
Duration: 3FT Hon

Entry Requirements: *Foundation:* Merit. *GCE:* 180-240. *IB:* 26. *BTEC NC:* DM. *BTEC ND:* MMP.

CF6V BSc Sport & Exercise Science and Geography
Duration: 3FT Hon

Entry Requirements: *Foundation:* Merit. *GCE:* 180-240. *IB:* 26. *BTEC NC:* DM. *BTEC ND:* MMP.

CF6P BSc Sport & Exercise Science and Geology
Duration: 3FT Hon

Entry Requirements: *Foundation:* Merit. *GCE:* 180-240. *IB:* 26. *BTEC NC:* DM. *BTEC ND:* MMP.

CCQV BSc Sport & Exercise Science and Psychology
Duration: 3FT Hon

Entry Requirements: *Foundation:* Merit. *GCE:* 180-240. *IB:* 26. *BTEC NC:* DM. *BTEC ND:* MMP.

CL69 BSc Sport & Exercise Science and Third World Development
Duration: 3FT Hon

Entry Requirements: *Foundation:* Merit. *GCE:* 180-240. *IB:* 26. *BTEC NC:* DM. *BTEC ND:* MMP.

CGQ4 BSc Sport & Exercise Science and Web-based Systems
Duration: 3FT Hon

Entry Requirements: *Foundation:* Merit. *GCE:* 180-240. *IB:* 26. *BTEC NC:* DM. *BTEC ND:* MMP.

CC63 BSc Sport & Exercise Science and Zoology

Duration: 3FT Hon

Entry Requirements: *Foundation:* Merit. *GCE:* 180-240. *IB:* 26. *BTEC NC:* DM. *BTEC ND:* MMP.

CC61 BSc Sport & Exercise Studies and Biology

Duration: 3FT Hon

Entry Requirements: *Foundation:* Merit. *GCE:* 180-240. *IB:* 26. *BTEC NC:* DM. *BTEC ND:* MMP.

CG61 BSc Sport & Exercise Studies and Mathematics

Duration: 3FT Hon

Entry Requirements: *Foundation:* Merit. *GCE:* 180-240. *IB:* 26. *BTEC NC:* DM. *BTEC ND:* MMP.

CW62 BSc/BA Sport & Exercise Science and Creative Design Practice

Duration: 3FT Hon

Entry Requirements: *GCE:* 180-240. *BTEC NC:* DM. *BTEC ND:* MMP.

CX6H BSc/BA Sport & Exercise Science and Education Studies

Duration: 3FT Hon

Entry Requirements: *Foundation:* Merit. *GCE:* 180-240. *IB:* 26. *BTEC NC:* DM. *BTEC ND:* MMP.

E28 UNIVERSITY OF EAST LONDON

DOCKLANDS CAMPUS
UNIVERSITY WAY
LONDON E16 2RD

t: 020 8223 2835 f: 020 8223 2978
e: admiss@uel.ac.uk
// www.uel.ac.uk

W4CP BA Theatre Studies with Sports & Exercise Science

Duration: 3FT Hon

Entry Requirements: *GCE:* 200. *IB:* 24. *BTEC NC:* DM. *BTEC ND:* MMP. *OCR ND:* Merit. *OCR NED:* Pass.

C7C6 BSc Biochemistry with Sports & Exercise Science

Duration: 3FT Hon

Entry Requirements: *GCE:* 200. *IB:* 24. *BTEC NC:* DM. *BTEC ND:* MMP. *OCR ND:* Merit. *OCR NED:* Pass.

C600 BSc Sport and Exercise Science

Duration: 3FT Hon

Entry Requirements: *GCE:* 80.

C601 BSc Sport and Exercise Science (Extended)

Duration: 4FT Hon

Entry Requirements: *GCE:* 80.

C6BC BSc Sports & Exercise Science with Human Biology

Duration: 3FT Hon

Entry Requirements: *GCE:* 200. *IB:* 24. *BTEC NC:* DM. *BTEC ND:* MMP.

C6CV BSc Sports & Exercise Science with Psychology

Duration: 3FT Hon

Entry Requirements: *GCE:* 200. *IB:* 24.

E42 EDGE HILL UNIVERSITY

ORMSKIRK
LANCASHIRE L39 4QP

t: 0800 195 5063 f: 01695 584355
e: enquiries@edgehill.ac.uk
// www.edgehill.ac.uk

C602 BSc Sport and Exercise Science

Duration: 3FT Hon

Entry Requirements: *GCE:* 240. *IB:* 28. *BTEC NC:* DD. *BTEC ND:* MMM. *OCR ND:* Distinction.

E56 THE UNIVERSITY OF EDINBURGH

STUDENT RECRUITMENT & ADMISSIONS
57 GEORGE SQUARE
EDINBURGH EH8 9JU

t: 0131 650 4360 f: 0131 651 1236
e: sra.enquiries@ed.ac.uk
// www.ed.ac.uk/studying/undergraduate/

C610 BSc Applied Sport Science

Duration: 4FT Hon

Entry Requirements: *GCE:* BBC. *SQAH:* BBBB. *IB:* 32.

E59 EDINBURGH NAPIER UNIVERSITY

CRAIGLOCKHART CAMPUS
EDINBURGH EH14 1DJ

t: +44 (0)8452 60 60 40 f: 0131 455 6464
e: info@napier.ac.uk
// www.napier.ac.uk

C8C6 BSc Psychology with Sport & Exercise Science

Duration: 3FT/4FT Ord/Hon

Entry Requirements: *GCE:* 230.

CB69 BSc Sport & Exercise Science (Sports Coaching top up)
Duration: 1FT Ord

Entry Requirements: Contact the institution for details.

CX61 BSc Sport & Exercise Science (Sports Coaching)
Duration: 3FT/4FT Ord/Hon

Entry Requirements: *GCE:* 260.

C601 BSc Sport & Exercise Science (top-up)
Duration: 1FT Ord

Entry Requirements: *GCE:* 240.

C600 BSc Sport and Exercise Science
Duration: 3FT/4FT Ord/Hon

Entry Requirements: *GCE:* 240.

CC68 BSc Sport and Exercise Science (Sport Psychology)
Duration: 3FT/4FT Ord/Hon

Entry Requirements: *GCE:* 260.

C602 BSc Sports Technology
Duration: 3FT/4FT Ord/Hon

Entry Requirements: *GCE:* 220.

E70 THE UNIVERSITY OF ESSEX
WIVENHOE PARK
COLCHESTER
ESSEX CO4 3SQ

t: 01206 873666 **f:** 01206 873423
e: admit@essex.ac.uk

// www.essex.ac.uk

CC16 BSc Sports Science and Biology
Duration: 3FT Hon

Entry Requirements: *GCE:* 280 - 320. *SQAH:* AABB-BBBB. *BTEC NC:* DM. *BTEC ND:* DMM. *OCR ND:* Distinction.

F66 FARNBOROUGH COLLEGE OF TECHNOLOGY
BOUNDARY ROAD
FARNBOROUGH
HAMPSHIRE GU14 6SB

t: 01252 407028 **f:** 01252 407041
e: admissions@farn-ct.ac.uk

// www.farn-ct.ac.uk

C601 BSc Sport Science (Exercise and Health Management)
Duration: 3FT Hon

Entry Requirements: Contact the institution for details.

G14 UNIVERSITY OF GLAMORGAN, CARDIFF AND PONTYPRIDD
ENQUIRIES AND ADMISSIONS UNIT
PONTYPRIDD CF37 1DL

t: 0800 716925 **f:** 01443 654050
e: enquiries@glam.ac.uk

// www.glam.ac.uk

CC61 BSc Biology and Sports Science
Duration: 3FT Hon

Entry Requirements: *GCE:* 200-240. *IB:* 28. *BTEC NC:* DM. *BTEC ND:* MMP.

C1C6 BSc Biology with Sports Science
Duration: 3FT Hon

Entry Requirements: *GCE:* 180-220. *IB:* 28. *BTEC NC:* DM. *BTEC ND:* MMP.

C600 BSc Sport and Exercise Science
Duration: 3FT/4SW Hon

Entry Requirements: *GCE:* 200-240. *IB:* 28. *BTEC NC:* DM. *BTEC ND:* MMP.

C605 BSc Sports Science and Rugby
Duration: 3FT Hon

Entry Requirements: *GCE:* 200-240. *IB:* 28. *BTEC NC:* DM. *BTEC ND:* MMP.

C6C1 BSc Sports Science with Biology
Duration: 3FT Hon

Entry Requirements: *GCE:* 180-220. *IB:* 26. *BTEC NC:* DM. *BTEC ND:* MMP.

G50 THE UNIVERSITY OF GLOUCESTERSHIRE
HARDWICK CAMPUS
ST PAUL'S ROAD
CHELTENHAM GL50 4BS

t: 01242 714501 **f:** 01242 543334
e: admissions@glos.ac.uk

// www.glos.ac.uk

C600 BSc Sport & Exercise Sciences
Duration: 3FT Hon

Entry Requirements: *GCE:* 200-280.

C603 BSc Sport Science
Duration: 3FT Hon

Entry Requirements: *GCE:* 240-280.

C609 BSc Sport Science
Duration: 2FT Hon

Entry Requirements: *GCE:* 200-300.

C608 BSc Sport Science and Sports Development

Duration: 3FT Hon

Entry Requirements: *GCE:* 200-280.

C611 BSc Sports Strength & Conditioning

Duration: 3FT Hon

Entry Requirements: *GCE:* 200-280.

C612 BSc Sports Strength & Conditioning and Sport Science

Duration: 3FT Hon

Entry Requirements: *GCE:* 200-280.

G53 GLYNDWR UNIVERSITY

PLAS COCH
MOLD ROAD
WREXHAM LL11 2AW
t: 01978 293439 f: 01978 290008
e: SID@glyndwr.ac.uk
// www.glyndwr.ac.uk

C606 BSc Sport and Exercise Sciences

Duration: 3FT Hon

Entry Requirements: *GCE:* 240.

G70 UNIVERSITY OF GREENWICH

GREENWICH CAMPUS
OLD ROYAL NAVAL COLLEGE
PARK ROW
LONDON SE10 9LS
t: 0800 005 006 f: 020 8331 8145
e: courseinfo@gre.ac.uk
// www.gre.ac.uk

C600 BSc Sports Science

Duration: 3FT Hon

Entry Requirements: *GCE:* 180. *IB:* 24.

C6N6 BSc Sports Science with Human Resource Management

Duration: 3FT Hon

Entry Requirements: *GCE:* 180. *IB:* 24.

C690 BSc Sports Science with Professional Football Coaching

Duration: 3FT Hon

Entry Requirements: *GCE:* 180. *IB:* 24.

C6R4 BSc Sports Science with Spanish

Duration: 3FT Hon

Entry Requirements: *GCE:* 180. *IB:* 24.

C604 FdSc Sports Science

Duration: 2FT Fdg

Entry Requirements: Contact the institution for details.

C6XC FdSc Sports Science with Coaching

Duration: 2FT Fdg

Entry Requirements: Contact the institution for details.

C602 FdSc Sports Science, Fitness and Health

Duration: 2FT Hon

Entry Requirements: Contact the institution for details.

006C HND Sports Science

Duration: 2FT HND

Entry Requirements: *GCE:* 40. *IB:* 24.

H24 HERIOT-WATT UNIVERSITY, EDINBURGH

EDINBURGH CAMPUS
EDINBURGH EH14 4AS
t: 0131 449 5111 f: 0131 451 3630
e: ugadmissions@hw.ac.uk
// www.hw.ac.uk

C600 BSc Sport and Exercise Science

Duration: 4FT Hon

Entry Requirements: *GCE:* CCC. *SQAH:* BBBB. *SQAAH:* BBB. *IB:* 30.

C6C8 BSc Sport and Exercise Science with Psychology

Duration: 4FT Hon

Entry Requirements: *GCE:* CCC. *SQAH:* BBBB. *SQAAH:* BBB. *IB:* 30.

H72 THE UNIVERSITY OF HULL

THE UNIVERSITY OF HULL
COTTINGHAM ROAD
HULL HU6 7RX
t: 01482 466100 f: 01482 442290
e: admissions@hull.ac.uk
// www.hull.ac.uk

C601 BSc Sport and Exercise Science

Duration: 3FT Hon

Entry Requirements: *GCE:* 240-280. *IB:* 30.

K24 THE UNIVERSITY OF KENT

INFORMATION, RECRUITMENT & ADMISSIONS
REGISTRY
UNIVERSITY OF KENT
CANTERBURY. KENT CT2 7NZ

t: 01227 827272 f: 01227 827077
e: information@kent.ac.uk
// www.kent.ac.uk

C602 BSc Sport, Exercise & Fitness Science (Training and Fitness)

Duration: 3FT Hon

Entry Requirements: *GCE:* 240. *SQAH:* ABBCC. *IB:* 27. *BTEC NC:* DD. *BTEC ND:* MMM. *OCR ND:* Distinction.

K84 KINGSTON UNIVERSITY

STUDENT INFORMATION & ADVICE CENTRE
COOPER HOUSE
40-46 SURBITON ROAD
KINGSTON UPON THAMES KT1 2HX

t: 020 8547 7053 f: 020 8547 7080
e: aps@kingston.ac.uk
// www.kingston.ac.uk

CCD6 BSc Biology and Sports Science (Foundation)

Duration: 4FT Hon

Entry Requirements: *GCE:* 40.

CC1P BSc Human Biology and Sports Science

Duration: 3FT Hon

Entry Requirements: *GCE:* 200-280.

C6ND BSc Sport Science with Business (Foundation)

Duration: 4FT Hon

Entry Requirements: *GCE:* 40.

C601 BSc Sports Science

Duration: 4SW Hon

Entry Requirements: *GCE:* 220-280.

C602 BSc Sports Science

Duration: 4FT Hon

Entry Requirements: *GCE:* 40.

C6MC BSc Sports Science with Law

Duration: 3FT Hon

Entry Requirements: *GCE:* 220-280.

L51 LIVERPOOL JOHN MOORES UNIVERSITY

ROSCOE COURT
4 RODNEY STREET
LIVERPOOL L1 2TZ

t: 0151 231 5090 f: 0151 231 3462
e: recruitment@ljmu.ac.uk
// www.ljmu.ac.uk

C600 BSc Sports Science

Duration: 3FT Hon

Entry Requirements: *GCE:* 280-300. *IB:* 28.

L68 LONDON METROPOLITAN UNIVERSITY

166-220 HOLLOWAY ROAD
LONDON N7 8DB

t: 020 7133 4200
e: admissions@londonmet.ac.uk
// www.londonmet.ac.uk

CC16 BA/BSc Biological Sciences and Sports Science

Duration: 3FT Hon

Entry Requirements: *GCE:* 200. *IB:* 28.

FC16 BA/BSc Chemistry and Sports Science

Duration: 3FT Hon

Entry Requirements: *GCE:* 200. *IB:* 28.

DC66 BA/BSc Consumer Studies and Sports Science

Duration: 3FT Hon

Entry Requirements: *GCE:* 200. *IB:* 28.

NC26 BA/BSc Sports Management and Sports Science

Duration: 3FT Hon

Entry Requirements: *GCE:* 200. *IB:* 28.

FC46 BSc Forensic Science and Sports Science

Duration: 3FT Hon

Entry Requirements: *GCE:* 180. *IB:* 28.

LC46 BSc Health Studies and Sports Science

Duration: 3FT Hon

Entry Requirements: *GCE:* 200. *IB:* 28.

C603 BSc Sports Science

Duration: 3FT Hon

Entry Requirements: *GCE:* 200. *IB:* 28.

C601 BSc Sports Science & Coaching

Duration: 3FT/4SW Hon

Entry Requirements: *GCE:* 160. *IB:* 28.

L75 LONDON SOUTH BANK UNIVERSITY

103 BOROUGH ROAD
LONDON SE1 0AA
t: 020 7815 7815 f: 020 7815 8273
e: enquiry@lsbu.ac.uk
// www.lsbu.ac.uk

C600 BSc Sport and Exercise Science

Duration: 3FT Hon

Entry Requirements: *GCE:* 160. *IB:* 24. *BTEC NC:* MM. *BTEC ND:* MPP.

C602 BSc Sports and Exercise Science

Duration: 1.5FT Hon

Entry Requirements: HND required.

C601 FdSc Sport and Exercise Science

Duration: 2FT Fdg

Entry Requirements: *GCE:* 80.

L77 LOUGHBOROUGH COLLEGE

RADMOOR ROAD
LOUGHBOROUGH LE11 3BT
t: 0845 166 2950 f: 0845 833 2840
e: info@loucoll.ac.uk
// www.loucoll.ac.uk

C601 BSc Applied Sports Science (top-up)

Duration: 1FT Hon

Entry Requirements: *GCE:* 80.

006C HND Sport and Exercise Science

Duration: 2FT HND

Entry Requirements: *GCE:* 40.

L79 LOUGHBOROUGH UNIVERSITY

LOUGHBOROUGH
LEICESTERSHIRE LE11 3TU
t: 01509 223522 f: 01509 223905
e: admissions@lboro.ac.uk
// www.lboro.ac.uk

QC36 BA English and Sports Science

Duration: 3FT Hon

Entry Requirements: *GCE:* 340. *SQAH:* BBBCCC. *SQAAH:* AB-BB. *IB:* 34.

FCC6 BSc Chemistry and Sports Science (4 year SW)

Duration: 4SW Hon

Entry Requirements: *GCE:* 300. *SQAH:* BBBB. *SQAAH:* BB. *IB:* 34. *BTEC ND:* DMM.

FC86 BSc Geography and Sports Science

Duration: 3FT Hon

Entry Requirements: *GCE:* 320-340. *IB:* 34. *BTEC ND:* DDM.

GC16 BSc Mathematics and Sports Science (4 year SW)

Duration: 4SW Hon

Entry Requirements: *GCE:* 340. *IB:* 30. *BTEC ND:* DDM.

CX63 BSc Sport and Exercise Science

Duration: 3FT Hon

Entry Requirements: *GCE:* 360. *IB:* 34. *BTEC ND:* DDD.

FC36 BSc Sports Science and Physics

Duration: 3FT Hon

Entry Requirements: *GCE:* 300. *SQAH:* BBCCC. *SQAAH:* BB. *IB:* 30. *BTEC ND:* DMM.

CF63 BSc Sports Science and Physics (4 year SW)

Duration: 4SW Hon

Entry Requirements: *GCE:* 300. *SQAH:* BBCCC. *SQAAH:* BB. *IB:* 30. *BTEC ND:* DMM.

CN62 BSc Sports Science with Management

Duration: 3FT Hon

Entry Requirements: *GCE:* 320-340. *IB:* 30. *BTEC ND:* DDD.

M40 THE MANCHESTER METROPOLITAN UNIVERSITY

ADMISSIONS OFFICE
ALL SAINTS (GMS)
ALL SAINTS
MANCHESTER M15 6BH
t: 0161 247 2000
// www.mmu.ac.uk

C602 BSc Sport and Exercise Science (Foundation)

Duration: 4FT Hon

Entry Requirements: Contact the institution for details.

M80 MIDDLESEX UNIVERSITY

MIDDLESEX UNIVERSITY
THE BURROUGHS
LONDON NW4 4BT

t: 020 8411 5555 f: 020 8411 5649
e: enquiries@mdx.ac.uk

// www.mdx.ac.uk

C603 BSc Sport and Exercise Science (Clinical Exercise)

Duration: 3FT Hon

Entry Requirements: *GCE:* 200-300. *IB:* 28.

CC68 BSc Sport and Exercise Science (Sport and Exercise Psychology)

Duration: 3FT Hon

Entry Requirements: *GCE:* 200-300. *IB:* 28.

M99 MYERSCOUGH COLLEGE

MYERSCOUGH HALL
BILSBORROW
PRESTON PR3 0RY

t: 01995 642222 f: 01995 642333
e: enquiries@myerscough.ac.uk

// www.myerscough.ac.uk

C600 FdSc Sport & Exercise Science

Duration: 2FT Fdg

Entry Requirements: *GCE:* A-C. *SQAH:* AA-CC. *SQAAH:* A-C. *IB:* 24. *BTEC NC:* PP. *BTEC ND:* PPP.

N49 NESCOT, SURREY

REIGATE ROAD
EWELL
EPSOM
SURREY KT17 3DS

t: 020 8394 3038 f: 020 8394 3030
e: info@nescot.ac.uk

// www.nescot.ac.uk

006C HND Sports and Exercise Sciences

Duration: 1FT/2FT HNC/HND

Entry Requirements: *GCE:* DD. *BTEC ND:* PPP.

N91 NOTTINGHAM TRENT UNIVERSITY

DRYDEN CENTRE
BURTON STREET
NOTTINGHAM NG1 4BU

t: +44 (0) 115 941 8418 f: +44 (0) 115 848 6063
e: admissions@ntu.ac.uk

// www.ntu.ac.uk/

CG6C BSc Sport Science and Mathematics

Duration: 3FT Hon

Entry Requirements: *GCE:* 240. *IB:* 26. *BTEC NC:* DD. *BTEC ND:* MMM.

O66 OXFORD BROOKES UNIVERSITY

ADMISSIONS OFFICE
HEADINGTON CAMPUS
GIPSY LANE
OXFORD OX3 0BP

t: 01865 483040 f: 01865 483983
e: admissions@brookes.ac.uk

// www.brookes.ac.uk

CC6V BA/BSc Sport & Exercise Science/Psychology

Duration: 3FT Hon

Entry Requirements: *GCE:* BBB.

CC1P BA/BSc Sports Science/Biology

Duration: 3FT Hon

Entry Requirements: *GCE:* BBC.

CC8P BA/BSc Sports Science/Psychology

Duration: 3FT Hon

Entry Requirements: *GCE:* BBB.

C604 BA/BSc Sports Science/Sports & Coaching Studies

Duration: 3FT Hon

Entry Requirements: *GCE:* BBC.

CCX6 BSc Biological Sciences/Sports Science

Duration: 3FT Hon

Entry Requirements: *GCE:* BBC.

CC61 BSc Sport & Exercise Science/Biology

Duration: 3FT Hon

Entry Requirements: *GCE:* BBC.

CC6C BSc Sport & Exercise Science/Ecology

Duration: 3FT Hon

Entry Requirements: *GCE:* BCC.

C601 BSc Sport and Exercise Science
Duration: 3FT Hon

Entry Requirements: *GCE:* BBC.

C602 BSc Sports Science
Duration: 3FT Hon

Entry Requirements: *GCE:* BBC.

CC1Q BSc Sports Science/Ecology
Duration: 3FT Hon

Entry Requirements: *GCE:* BCC.

BC1P BSc Sports Science/Human Biology
Duration: 3FT Hon

Entry Requirements: *GCE:* BBC.

P60 UNIVERSITY OF PLYMOUTH
DRAKE CIRCUS
PLYMOUTH PL4 8AA

t: 01752 588037 f: 01752 588050
e: admissions@plymouth.ac.uk

// www.plymouth.ac.uk

CJ69 BSc Applied Marine Sport Science
Duration: 3FT Hon

Entry Requirements: *GCE:* 200.

P63 UCP MARJON - UNIVERSITY COLLEGE PLYMOUTH ST MARK & ST JOHN
DERRIFORD ROAD
PLYMOUTH PL6 8BH

t: 01752 636890 f: 01752 636819
e: admissions@marjon.ac.uk

// www.ucpmarjon.ac.uk

C6X3 BA Applied Sports Science & Coaching with Education Studies
Duration: 3FT Hon

Entry Requirements: *GCE:* 240.

C604 BA Applied Sports Science & Coaching with Outdoor Adventure
Duration: 3FT Hon

Entry Requirements: *GCE:* 240.

C600 BA Outdoor Adventure with Applied Sports Science & Coaching
Duration: 3FT Hon

Entry Requirements: *GCE:* 180.

CX61 BSc Applied Sports Science & Coaching
Duration: 3FT Hon

Entry Requirements: *GCE:* 220.

P80 UNIVERSITY OF PORTSMOUTH
ACADEMIC REGISTRY
UNIVERSITY HOUSE
WINSTON CHURCHILL AVENUE
PORTSMOUTH PO1 2UP

t: 023 9284 8484 f: 023 9284 3082
e: admissions@port.ac.uk

// www.port.ac.uk

C601 BSc Water Sports Science
Duration: 3FT Hon

Entry Requirements: *GCE:* 200.

R48 ROEHAMPTON UNIVERSITY
ERASMUS HOUSE
ROEHAMPTON LANE
LONDON SW15 5PU

t: 020 8392 3232 f: 020 8392 3470
e: enquiries@roehampton.ac.uk

// www.roehampton.ac.uk

C602 BSc Sport and Exercise Sciences
Duration: 3FT Hon

Entry Requirements: *GCE:* 240-280. *IB:* 24. *BTEC NC:* DD. *BTEC ND:* MMM. *OCR ND:* Distinction. *OCR NED:* Merit.

GC46 BSc/BA Computing Studies and Sport Science
Duration: 3FT Hon

Entry Requirements: *GCE:* 240-280. *IB:* 24. *BTEC NC:* DD. *BTEC ND:* MMM. *OCR ND:* Distinction. *OCR NED:* Merit.

S03 THE UNIVERSITY OF SALFORD
SALFORD M5 4WT

t: 0161 295 4545 f: 0161 295 3126
e: ugadmissions-exrel@salford.ac.uk

// www.salford.ac.uk

C610 BSc Applied Sports Science
Duration: 3FT Hon

Entry Requirements: *GCE:* 240. *SQAH:* BCCCC. *SQAAH:* CCC. *IB:* 24. *BTEC NC:* DD. *BTEC ND:* MMM.

S26 SOLIHULL COLLEGE

BLOSSOMFIELD ROAD
SOLIHULL
WEST MIDLANDS B91 1SB

t: 0121 678 7247 f: 0121 678 7200
e: enquiries@solihull.ac.uk

// www.solihull.ac.uk

006C HND Sport & Exercise Science

Duration: 2FT HND

Entry Requirements: *GCE:* 180.

S30 SOUTHAMPTON SOLENT UNIVERSITY

EAST PARK TERRACE
SOUTHAMPTON
HAMPSHIRE SO14 0RT

t: +44 (0) 23 8031 9039 f: + 44 (0)23 8022 2259
e: admissions@solent.ac.uk or ask@solent.ac.uk

// www.solent.ac.uk/

C602 BSc Applied Sport Science

Duration: 3FT Hon

Entry Requirements: *GCE:* 40.

S64 ST MARY'S UNIVERSITY COLLEGE, TWICKENHAM

WALDEGRAVE ROAD
STRAWBERRY HILL
MIDDLESEX TW1 4SX

t: 020 8240 4029 f: 020 8240 2361
e: admit@smuc.ac.uk

// www.smuc.ac.uk

CXP3 BA/BSc Education & Employment and Sport Science

Duration: 3FT Hon

Entry Requirements: *GCE:* 160-200. *BTEC NC:* MM. *BTEC ND:* MPP.

QC56 BA/BSc Irish Studies and Sport Science

Duration: 3FT Hon

Entry Requirements: *GCE:* 160-200. *BTEC NC:* MM. *BTEC ND:* MPP.

CN62 BA/BSc Management Studies and Sport Science

Duration: 3FT Hon

Entry Requirements: *GCE:* 160-200. *BTEC NC:* MM. *BTEC ND:* MPP.

CV65 BA/BSc Philosophy and Sport Science

Duration: 3FT Hon

Entry Requirements: *GCE:* 160-200. *BTEC NC:* MM. *BTEC ND:* MPP.

CW68 BA/BSc Professional & Creative Writing and Sport Science

Duration: 3FT Hon

Entry Requirements: *GCE:* 160-200. *BTEC NC:* MM. *BTEC ND:* MPP.

C6Q5 BA/BSc Sport Science with Irish Studies

Duration: 3FT Hon

Entry Requirements: *GCE:* 160-200. *BTEC NC:* MM. *BTEC ND:* MPP.

MC26 BSc Business Law and Sport Science

Duration: 3FT Hon

Entry Requirements: Contact the institution for details.

CC86 BSc Psychology and Sport Science

Duration: 3FT Hon

Entry Requirements: *GCE:* 160-200. *BTEC NC:* MM. *BTEC ND:* MPP.

S72 STAFFORDSHIRE UNIVERSITY

COLLEGE ROAD
STOKE ON TRENT ST4 2DE

t: 01782 292753 f: 01782 292740
e: admissions@staffs.ac.uk

// www.staffs.ac.uk

C601 BSc Sport and Exercise Science

Duration: 3FT Hon

Entry Requirements: *GCE:* 180-240. *IB:* 24. *BTEC NC:* DM. *BTEC ND:* MMM.

S75 THE UNIVERSITY OF STIRLING

STIRLING FK9 4LA

t: 01786 467044 f: 01786 466800
e: admissions@stir.ac.uk

// www.stir.ac.uk

CC61 BSc Sport and Exercise Science

Duration: 4FT Hon

Entry Requirements: *GCE:* BCC. *SQAH:* BBBB. *SQAAH:* AAA-CCC. *BTEC ND:* DMM.

S82 UNIVERSITY CAMPUS SUFFOLK

WATERFRONT BUILDING
NEPTUNE QUAY
IPSWICH
SUFFOLK IP4 1QJ

t: 01473 338348 f: 01473 339900
e: info@ucs.ac.uk

// www.ucs.ac.uk

C600 BSc Sport & Exercise Science

Duration: 3FT Hon

Entry Requirements: *GCE:* 200. *IB:* 24. *BTEC NC:* MP. *BTEC ND:* PPP.

S84 UNIVERSITY OF SUNDERLAND
STUDENT HELPLINE
THE STUDENT GATEWAY
CHESTER ROAD
SUNDERLAND SR1 3SD

t: 0191 515 3000 f: 0191 515 3805
e: student-helpline@sunderland.ac.uk
// www.sunderland.ac.uk

C608 BA Sport Sciences (Foundation) (4 years)
Duration: 4FT/5SW Hon

Entry Requirements: *GCE:* 100-360. *SQAH:* CC.

T40 THAMES VALLEY UNIVERSITY
ST MARY'S ROAD
EALING
LONDON W5 5RF

t: 0800 036 8888 f: 020 8566 1353
e: learning.advice@tvu.ac.uk
// www.tvu.ac.uk

CB6X BSc Sports and Exercise Science
Duration: 3FT Hon

Entry Requirements: *GCE:* 200. *IB:* 28. Interview required.

T85 TRURO AND PENWITH COLLEGE (FORMERLY TRURO COLLEGE)
TRURO COLLEGE
COLLEGE ROAD
TRURO
CORNWALL TR1 3XX

t: 01872 267122 f: 01872 267526
e: heinfo@trurocollege.ac.uk
// www.trurocollege.ac.uk

C602 FdSc Sports Science and Injury Management
Duration: 2FT Fdg

Entry Requirements: *GCE:* 60. *IB:* 24. *BTEC NC:* PP. *BTEC ND:* PPP.

U20 UNIVERSITY OF ULSTER
COLERAINE
CO. LONDONDERRY
NORTHERN IRELAND BT52 1SA

t: 028 7032 4221 f: 028 7032 4908
e: online@ulster.ac.uk
// www.ulster.ac.uk

C600 BSc Sport and Exercise Sciences
Duration: 3FT Hon

Entry Requirements: *GCE:* ABB. *SQAH:* AAABC. *SQAAH:* ABB. *IB:* 26. *BTEC ND:* DDM.

W12 WALSALL COLLEGE
WALSALL COLLEGE
LITTLETON STREET WEST
WALSALL WS2 8ES

t: 01922 657000 f: 01922 657083
e: ckemp@walsallcollege.ac.uk
// www.walsallcollege.ac.uk

006C HND Sport and Exercise Science
Duration: 2FT HND

Entry Requirements: Interview required.

W25 WARWICKSHIRE COLLEGE
WARWICK NEW ROAD
LEAMINGTON SPA
WARWICKSHIRE CV32 5JE

t: 01926 318 000 f: 01926 318 111
e: he@warkscol.ac.uk
// www.warkscol.ac.uk

DC36 BSc Sports Science (Equine and Human)
Duration: 3FT/4SW Hon

Entry Requirements: *GCE:* 180. *IB:* 28. *BTEC ND:* MPP.

DC4P FdSc Sports Science (Equine and Human)
Duration: 2FT/3SW Fdg

Entry Requirements: *GCE:* 80.

106C HND Sport and Exercise Sciences (Sport Therapy)
Duration: 2FT HND

Entry Requirements: *GCE:* 80. *BTEC ND:* PPP.

W75 UNIVERSITY OF WOLVERHAMPTON
ADMISSIONS UNIT
MX207, CAMP STREET
WOLVERHAMPTON
WEST MIDLANDS WV1 1AD

t: 01902 321000 f: 01902 321896
e: admissions@wlv.ac.uk
// www.wlv.ac.uk

BC96 BSc Health Studies and Sport & Exercise Science
Duration: 3FT Hon

Entry Requirements: *GCE:* 160-220. *IB:* 30.

CN61 BSc Sport & Exercise Science and Business
Duration: 3FT Hon

Entry Requirements: *GCE:* 220. *IB:* 28. *BTEC NC:* DD. *BTEC ND:* MMM.

W76 UNIVERSITY OF WINCHESTER

WINCHESTER
HANTS SO22 4NR

t: 01962 827234 f: 01962 827288
e: course.enquiries@winchester.ac.uk

// www.winchester.ac.uk

C602 BSc Sports Science

Duration: 3FT Hon

Entry Requirements: *Foundation:* Distinction. *GCE:* 240-280. *IB:* 24.
BTEC NC: DD. *BTEC ND:* MMM. *OCR ND:* Distinction.

C603 DipHE Sports Science

Duration: 2FT Dip

Entry Requirements: *Foundation:* Pass. *GCE:* 120. *IB:* 20. *BTEC NC:*
MP. *BTEC ND:* PPP.

Y75 YORK ST JOHN UNIVERSITY

LORD MAYOR'S WALK
YORK YO31 7EX

t: 01904 876598 f: 01904 876940/876921
e: admissions@yorksj.ac.uk

// www.yorksj.ac.uk

CB6X BSc Sports Science and Injury Management

Duration: 3FT Hon

Entry Requirements: Contact the institution for details.

SPORTS EXERCISE AND HEALTH

A20 THE UNIVERSITY OF ABERDEEN

UNIVERSITY OFFICE
KING'S COLLEGE
ABERDEEN AB24 3FX

t: +44 (0) 1224 273504 f: +44 (0) 1224 272034
e: sras@abdn.ac.uk

// www.abdn.ac.uk/sras

CX61 BSc Applied Sports Science and Education

Duration: 4FT Hon

Entry Requirements: Contact the institution for details.

XB19 BSc Education and Health Sciences

Duration: 4FT Hon

Entry Requirements: Contact the institution for details.

C603 BSc Sports Studies (Exercise and Health)

Duration: 4FT Hon

Entry Requirements: *GCE:* 240. *SQAH:* BBBB. *SQAAH:* BCC. *IB:* 28.
BTEC ND: MMM.

C602 MSci Sports and Exercise Science with Industrial Placement

Duration: 5FT Hon

Entry Requirements: *GCE:* 240. *SQAH:* BBBB. *SQAAH:* BCC. *IB:* 28.
BTEC ND: MMM.

C601 MSci Sports Studies (Exercise and Health) with Industrial Placement

Duration: 5FT Hon

Entry Requirements: *GCE:* 240. *SQAH:* BBBB. *SQAAH:* BCC. *IB:* 28.
BTEC ND: MMM.

A30 UNIVERSITY OF ABERTAY DUNDEE

BELL STREET
DUNDEE DD1 1HG

t: 01382 308080 f: 01382 308081
e: sro@abertay.ac.uk

// www.abertay.ac.uk

CN62 BA Sport and Management

Duration: 4FT Hon

Entry Requirements: *GCE:* DDD. *SQAH:* BBC. *IB:* 26. Interview
required.

CB64 BSc Sport & Exercise Nutrition

Duration: 4FT Hon

Entry Requirements: *GCE:* DDD. *SQAH:* BBC. *IB:* 26. Interview
required.

CC68 BSc Sport and Psychology

Duration: 4FT Hon

Entry Requirements: HND required.

A40 ABERYSTWYTH UNIVERSITY

WELCOME CENTRE, ABERYSTWYTH UNIVERSITY
PENGLAIS CAMPUS
ABERYSTWYTH
CEREDIGION SY23 3FB

t: 01970 622021 f: 01970 627410
e: ug-admissions@aber.ac.uk

// www.aber.ac.uk

CG65 BSc Sports and Information Technology

Duration: 3FT Hon

Entry Requirements: *GCE:* 240. *IB:* 24.

A44 ACCRINGTON & ROSSENDALE COLLEGE

BROAD OAK ROAD,
ACCRINGTON,
LANCASHIRE. BB5 2AW.

t: 01254 389933 **f:** 01254 354001
e: info@accross.ac.uk

// www.accross.ac.uk/

C600 FdA Physical Activity and Sport
Duration: 2FT Fdg

Entry Requirements: *BTEC ND:* MMM. Interview required.

B06 BANGOR UNIVERSITY

BANGOR
GWYNEDD LL57 2DG

t: 01248 382016/2017 **f:** 01248 370451
e: admissions@bangor.ac.uk

// www.bangor.ac.uk

CB69 BSc Sport, Health and Exercise Sciences.
Duration: 3FT Hon

Entry Requirements: *GCE:* 260-280. *IB:* 28.

B16 UNIVERSITY OF BATH

CLAVERTON DOWN
BATH BA2 7AY

t: 01225 383019 **f:** 01225 386366
e: admissions@bath.ac.uk

// www.bath.ac.uk

CHP3 MEng Sports Engineering (4 years)
Duration: 4FT Hon

Entry Requirements: *GCE:* AAA. *SQAAH:* AAA. *IB:* 36.

CHPH MEng Sports Engineering (5 year sandwich)
Duration: 5SW Hon

Entry Requirements: *GCE:* AAA. *SQAAH:* AAA. *IB:* 36.

C600 FdSc Sport (Health & Fitness)
Duration: 2FT Fdg

Entry Requirements: *GCE:* 80.

C601 FdSc Sport (Sports Performance)
Duration: 2FT Fdg

Entry Requirements: *GCE:* 120.

B22 UNIVERSITY OF BEDFORDSHIRE

PARK SQUARE
LUTON
BEDS LU1 3JU

t: 01582 489286 **f:** 01582 489323
e: admissions@beds.ac.uk

// www.beds.ac.uk

CN68 BA Sport and Adventure Recreation
Duration: 3FT Hon

Entry Requirements: Contact the institution for details.

CX69 BA Sport and Community Leadership
Duration: 3FT Hon

Entry Requirements: Contact the institution for details.

CN62 BA Sport Studies
Duration: 3FT Hon

Entry Requirements: *GCE:* 160-240. *SQAH:* BCC. *SQAAH:* BCC. *IB:* 30.

C612 BA Sports Studies
Duration: 3FT Hon

Entry Requirements: *GCE:* 180-220.

C610 BSc Sports Studies
Duration: 3FT Hon

Entry Requirements: *GCE:* 180-220.

B25 BIRMINGHAM CITY UNIVERSITY

PERRY BARR
BIRMINGHAM B42 2SU

t: 0121 331 5595 **f:** 0121 331 7994
e: choices@bcu.ac.uk

// www.bcu.ac.uk

BC96 BSc Health and Well-being (Exercise Science)
Duration: 3FT Hon

Entry Requirements: *GCE:* 200.

B41 BLACKPOOL AND THE FYLDE COLLEGE AN ASSOCIATE COLLEGE OF LANCASTER UNIVERSITY

ASHFIELD ROAD
BISPHAM
BLACKPOOL
LANCS FY2 0HB

t: 01253 504346 f: 01253 356127
e: admissions@blackpool.ac.uk

// www.blackpool.ac.uk

C601 BA Sports Development (Top-up)
Duration: 1FT Hon

Entry Requirements: HND required.

C600 FdA Sports Development
Duration: 2FT Fdg

Entry Requirements: GCE: 40. SQAH: C. SQAAH: C. BTEC NC: PP. BTEC ND: PPP.

B50 BOURNEMOUTH UNIVERSITY

TALBOT CAMPUS
FERN BARROW
POOLE
DORSET BH12 5BB

t: 01202 524111

// www.bournemouth.ac.uk

CB69 BSc Exercise Science (Health and Rehabilitation)
Duration: 3FT Hon

Entry Requirements: GCE: 240.

B70 BRIDGWATER COLLEGE

BATH ROAD
BRIDGWATER
SOMERSET TA6 4PZ

t: 01278 455464 f: 01278 444363
e: enquiries@bridgwater.ac.uk

// www.bridgwater.ac.uk

106C HND Sport and Exercise Sciences (Sports Science)
Duration: 2FT HND

Entry Requirements: GCE: 120.

B72 UNIVERSITY OF BRIGHTON

MITHRAS HOUSE
LEWES ROAD
BRIGHTON BN2 4AT

t: 01273 644644 f: 01273 642607
e: admissions@brighton.ac.uk

// www.brighton.ac.uk

C603 BA Sport Studies
Duration: 3FT Hon

Entry Requirements: GCE: BCC. IB: 30. BTEC ND: DMM.

C602 BSc Sport and Fitness (Top-up)
Duration: 1FT Hon

Entry Requirements: HND required.

C601 FdSc Sport and Fitness
Duration: 2FT Fdg

Entry Requirements: GCE: 80. IB: 24.

B80 UNIVERSITY OF THE WEST OF ENGLAND, BRISTOL

FRENCHAY CAMPUS
COLDHARBOUR LANE
BRISTOL BS16 1QY

t: +44 (0)117 32 83333 f: +44 (0)117 32 82810
e: admissions@uwe.ac.uk

// www.uwe.ac.uk

NCF6 BA Sports Business Management
Duration: 3FT Hon

Entry Requirements: GCE: 200-240.

CN62 FdA Sport and Exercise Management
Duration: 2FT Fdg

Entry Requirements: GCE: 120-160.

B84 BRUNEL UNIVERSITY

UXBRIDGE
MIDDLESEX UB8 3PH

t: 01895 265265 f: 01895 269790
e: admissions@brunel.ac.uk

// www.brunel.ac.uk

LC5P BA Youth Sport Work (JNC)
Duration: 3FT Hon

Entry Requirements: GCE: 320. IB: 28. BTEC ND: DMM.

C55 UNIVERSITY OF CHESTER

PARKGATE ROAD
CHESTER CH1 4BJ
t: 01244 511000 **f:** 01244 511300
e: enquiries@chester.ac.uk
// www.chester.ac.uk

NCM6 BA Advertising and Sport Development

Duration: 3FT Hon

Entry Requirements: *Foundation:* Pass. *GCE:* 240. *SQAH:* BBBB. *IB:* 24. *BTEC NC:* DM. *BTEC ND:* MMM.

N5CP BA Advertising with Sport Development

Duration: 3FT Hon

Entry Requirements: *Foundation:* Pass. *GCE:* 240. *SQAH:* BBBB. *IB:* 24. *BTEC NC:* DM. *BTEC ND:* MMM.

CN62 BA Business Management and Sport Development

Duration: 3FT Hon

Entry Requirements: *GCE:* 240. *SQAH:* BBBB. *IB:* 24. *BTEC NC:* DM. *BTEC ND:* MMM.

N2CQ BA Business Management with Sport Development

Duration: 3FT Hon

Entry Requirements: *GCE:* 240. *SQAH:* BBBB. *IB:* 24. *BTEC NC:* DM. *BTEC ND:* MMM.

N1CQ BA Business with Sport & Exercise Sciences

Duration: 3FT Hon

Entry Requirements: *GCE:* 240. *SQAH:* BBBB. *IB:* 24. *BTEC NC:* DM. *BTEC ND:* MMM.

GC4P BA Computing and Sport Development

Duration: 3FT Hon

Entry Requirements: *GCE:* 240. *SQAH:* BBBB. *IB:* 24. *BTEC NC:* DM. *BTEC ND:* MMM.

WC66 BA Digital Photography and Sport Development

Duration: 3FT Hon

Entry Requirements: *GCE:* 240. *SQAH:* BBBB. *IB:* 24. *BTEC NC:* DM. *BTEC ND:* MMM.

W6C6 BA Digital Photography with Sport Development

Duration: 3FT Hon

Entry Requirements: *GCE:* 240. *SQAH:* BBBB. *IB:* 24. *BTEC NC:* DM. *BTEC ND:* MMM.

NC86 BA Events Management and Sport Development

Duration: 3FT Hon

Entry Requirements: *GCE:* 240. *SQAH:* BBBB. *IB:* 24. *BTEC NC:* DM. *BTEC ND:* MMM.

N8C6 BA Events Management with Sport & Exercise Science

Duration: 3FT Hon

Entry Requirements: *GCE:* 240. *SQAH:* BBBB. *IB:* 24. *BTEC NC:* DM. *BTEC ND:* MMM.

N8CP BA Events Management with Sports Development

Duration: 3FT Hon

Entry Requirements: *GCE:* 240. *SQAH:* BBBB. *IB:* 24. *BTEC NC:* DM. *BTEC ND:* MMM.

R1C6 BA French with Sport & Exercise Science

Duration: 4FT Hon

Entry Requirements: *GCE:* 240. *SQAH:* BBBB. *IB:* 24. *BTEC NC:* DM. *BTEC ND:* MMM.

W2C6 BA Graphic Design with Sport Development

Duration: 3FT Hon

Entry Requirements: *GCE:* 240. *SQAH:* BBBB. *IB:* 24. *BTEC NC:* DM. *BTEC ND:* MMM.

N5CQ BA Marketing with Sport Development

Duration: 3FT Hon

Entry Requirements: *GCE:* 240. *SQAH:* BBBB. *IB:* 24. *BTEC NC:* DM. *BTEC ND:* MMM.

C602 BA Sport Development

Duration: 3FT Hon

Entry Requirements: *GCE:* 200 - 240. *SQAH:* BBBB. *IB:* 24. *BTEC NC:* DM. *BTEC ND:* MMM.

C6GL BA Sport Development with Computing

Duration: 3FT Hon

Entry Requirements: *GCE:* 240. *SQAH:* BBBB. *IB:* 24. *BTEC NC:* DM. *BTEC ND:* MMM.

C6W6 BA Sport Development with Digital Photography

Duration: 3FT Hon

Entry Requirements: *GCE:* 240. *SQAH:* BBBB. *IB:* 24. *BTEC NC:* DM. *BTEC ND:* MMM.

C6N8 BA Sport Development with Events Management

Duration: 3FT Hon

Entry Requirements: *GCE:* 240. *SQAH:* BBBB. *IB:* 24. *BTEC NC:* DM. *BTEC ND:* MMM.

C6NN BA Sport Development with Marketing

Duration: 3FT Hon

Entry Requirements: *GCE:* 240. *SQAH:* BBBB. *IB:* 24. *BTEC NC:* DM. *BTEC ND:* MMM.

G4CQ BSc Computing with Sport Development

Duration: 3FT Hon

Entry Requirements: *IB:* 24.

B4C6 BSc Nutrition with Sport & Exercise Sciences

Duration: 3FT Hon

Entry Requirements: *GCE:* 240. *SQAH:* BBBB. *IB:* 24. *BTEC NC:* DM. *BTEC ND:* MMM.

C6N2 BSc Sport & Exercise Sciences with Management

Duration: 3FT Hon

Entry Requirements: *GCE:* 240. *SQAH:* BBBB. *IB:* 24. *BTEC NC:* DM. *BTEC ND:* MMM.

C6G1 BSc Sport & Exercise Sciences with Mathematics

Duration: 3FT Hon

Entry Requirements: *GCE:* 240. *SQAH:* BBBB. *IB:* 24. *BTEC NC:* DM. *BTEC ND:* MPP.

C6C8 BSc Sport & Exercise Sciences with Psychology

Duration: 3FT Hon

Entry Requirements: *GCE:* 240. *SQAH:* BBBB. *IB:* 24. *BTEC NC:* DM. *BTEC ND:* MMM.

CB6X FdSc Fitness & Health

Duration: 2FT Fdg

Entry Requirements: *GCE:* 140. *SQAH:* CCCC. *IB:* 24.

C58 UNIVERSITY OF CHICHESTER

BISHOP OTTER CAMPUS
COLLEGE LANE
CHICHESTER
WEST SUSSEX PO19 6PE

t: 01243 816002 **f:** 01243 816161
e: admissions@chi.ac.uk

// www.chiuni.ac.uk

NC26 BA Sport and Fitness Management

Duration: 3FT Hon

Entry Requirements: *GCE:* 180-220. *IB:* 24. *BTEC NC:* DM. *BTEC ND:* MMP.

BC9P FdSc Health Promotion and Personal Training

Duration: 2FT Fdg

Entry Requirements: *GCE:* 80. *IB:* 24. *BTEC NC:* PP. *BTEC ND:* PPP. Interview required.

C69 CITY OF SUNDERLAND COLLEGE

BEDE CENTRE
DURHAM ROAD
SUNDERLAND SR3 4AH

t: 0191 511 6260 **f:** 0191 511 6380
e: highered.admissions@citysun.ac.uk

// www.citysun.ac.uk

CX6D FdSc Exercise Health and Fitness

Duration: 2FT Fdg

Entry Requirements: *GCE:* 80.

C85 COVENTRY UNIVERSITY

THE STUDENT CENTRE
COVENTRY UNIVERSITY
1 GULSON RD
COVENTRY CV1 2JH

t: 024 7615 2222 **f:** 024 7615 2223
e: studentenquiries@coventry.ac.uk

// www.coventry.ac.uk

C602 BSc Sport and Exercise Science (Sport Development)

Duration: 3FT Hon

Entry Requirements: *GCE:* 240. *BTEC NC:* DD. *BTEC ND:* MMM.

CB69 FdSc Exercise Science

Duration: 2FT Fdg

Entry Requirements: *GCE:* 80. *BTEC NC:* PP. *BTEC ND:* PPP.

006C HND Sport, Exercise and Therapy Sciences
Duration: 2FT HND

Entry Requirements: *GCE:* 60. *BTEC NC:* PP. *BTEC ND:* PPP.

C99 UNIVERSITY OF CUMBRIA
FUSEHILL STREET
CARLISLE
CUMBRIA CA1 2HH
t: 01228 616234 f: 01228 616235
// www.cumbria.ac.uk

C604 BA Coaching and Sport Development
Duration: 3FT Hon

Entry Requirements: *Foundation:* Distinction. *GCE:* 240. *IB:* 28. *BTEC NC:* DD. *BTEC ND:* MMM. *OCR ND:* Distinction.

C611 BA Sport Studies (Physical Activity and Sports Development)
Duration: 4SW Hon

Entry Requirements: Contact the institution for details.

C610 BSc Physical Activity and Health
Duration: 1FT Hon

Entry Requirements: Contact the institution for details.

C607 DipHE Sport Studies (Physical Activity &Sports Development)
Duration: 2FT Dip

Entry Requirements: *Foundation:* Pass. *GCE:* 80. *IB:* 24. *BTEC NC:* PP. *BTEC ND:* PPP.

C606 FdSc Physical Activity & Health
Duration: 2FT Fdg

Entry Requirements: *Foundation:* Pass. *GCE:* 40. *IB:* 30. *BTEC NC:* PP. *BTEC ND:* PPP. Interview required.

CN62 FdA Sport Development and Management
Duration: 2FT Fdg

Entry Requirements: Contact the institution for details.

D39 UNIVERSITY OF DERBY
KEDLESTON ROAD
DERBY DE22 1GB
t: 08701 202330 f: 01332 597724
e: askadmissions@derby.ac.uk
// www.derby.ac.uk

TC76 BA American Studies and Sport & Exercise Studies
Duration: 3FT Hon

Entry Requirements: *Foundation:* Merit. *GCE:* 180-240. *IB:* 26. *BTEC NC:* DM. *BTEC ND:* MMP.

WC86 BA Creative Writing and Sport & Exercise Studies
Duration: 3FT Hon

Entry Requirements: *Foundation:* Merit. *GCE:* 180-240. *IB:* 26. *BTEC NC:* DM. *BTEC ND:* MMP.

MC26 BA Criminology and Sport & Exercise Studies
Duration: 3FT Hon

Entry Requirements: *Foundation:* Merit. *GCE:* 180-240. *IB:* 26. *BTEC NC:* DM. *BTEC ND:* MMP.

WC56 BA Dance & Movement Studies and Sport & Exercise Studies
Duration: 3FT Hon

Entry Requirements: *Foundation:* Merit. *GCE:* 180-240. *IB:* 26. *BTEC NC:* DM. *BTEC ND:* MMP.

CNPV BA Martial Arts and Outdoor Recreation
Duration: 3FT Hon

Entry Requirements: *Foundation:* Merit. *GCE:* 160-240. *IB:* 26. *BTEC NC:* MM. *BTEC ND:* MMP.

C610 BA Martial Arts and Physical Activity & Health
Duration: 3FT Hon

Entry Requirements: *Foundation:* Merit. *GCE:* 160-240. *IB:* 26. *BTEC NC:* MM. *BTEC ND:* MMP.

NCVP BA Outdoor Recreation and Physical Activity & Health
Duration: 3FT Hon

Entry Requirements: *Foundation:* Merit. *GCE:* 160-240. *IB:* 26. *BTEC NC:* MM. *BTEC ND:* MMP.

NCVQ BA Outdoor Recreation and Sports Development
Duration: 3FT Hon

Entry Requirements: *Foundation:* Merit. *GCE:* 160-240. *IB:* 26. *BTEC NC:* MM. *BTEC ND:* MMP.

CNQW BA Physical Activity & Health and Adventure Tourism
Duration: 3FT Hon

Entry Requirements: *Foundation:* Merit. *GCE:* 160-240. *IB:* 26. *BTEC NC:* MM. *BTEC ND:* MMP.

NCWP BA Physical Activity & Health and Events Management
Duration: 3FT Hon

Entry Requirements: *Foundation:* Merit. *GCE:* 160-240. *IB:* 26. *BTEC NC:* MM. *BTEC ND:* MMP.

WC36 BA Popular Music Production and Sport & Exercise Studies

Duration: 3FT Hon

Entry Requirements: *Foundation:* Merit. *GCE:* 180-240. *IB:* 26. *BTEC NC:* DM. *BTEC ND:* MMP.

PC16 BA Public Services Management and Physical Activity & Health

Duration: 3FT Hon

Entry Requirements: *Foundation:* Merit. *GCE:* 160-240. *IB:* 26. *BTEC NC:* MM. *BTEC ND:* MMP.

CM61 BA Sport & Exercise Studies and Law

Duration: 3FT Hon

Entry Requirements: *Foundation:* Merit. *GCE:* 180-240. *IB:* 26. *BTEC NC:* DM. *BTEC ND:* MMP.

C605 BA Sport & Exercise Studies and Martial Arts Theory & Practice

Duration: 3FT Hon

Entry Requirements: *GCE:* 140-160. *IB:* 26. *BTEC NC:* MM. *BTEC ND:* MPP.

C609 BA Sports Development and Martial Arts Theory & Practice

Duration: 3FT Hon

Entry Requirements: *Foundation:* Merit. *GCE:* 160-240. *IB:* 26. *BTEC NC:* MM. *BTEC ND:* MMP.

CN68 BA Travel & Tourism and Sport & Exercise Studies

Duration: 3FT Hon

Entry Requirements: *Foundation:* Merit. *GCE:* 180-240. *IB:* 26. *BTEC NC:* DM. *BTEC ND:* MMP.

GC4P BA/BSc Computing Management and Sports & Exercise Studies

Duration: 3FT Hon

Entry Requirements: *Foundation:* Merit. *GCE:* 180-240. *IB:* 26. *BTEC NC:* DM. *BTEC ND:* MMP.

GC16 BA/BSc Mathematics and Sport & Exercise Studies

Duration: 3FT Hon

Entry Requirements: *Foundation:* Merit. *GCE:* 180-240. *IB:* 26. *BTEC NC:* DM. *BTEC ND:* MMP.

CNQF BA/BSc Sport & Exercise Science and Business Management

Duration: 3FT Hon

Entry Requirements: *Foundation:* Merit. *GCE:* 180-240. *IB:* 26. *BTEC NC:* DM. *BTEC ND:* MMP.

CL6X BA/BSc Sport & Exercise Studies and Third World Development

Duration: 3FT Hon

Entry Requirements: *Foundation:* Merit. *GCE:* 180-240. *IB:* 26. *BTEC NC:* DM. *BTEC ND:* MMP.

CC6H BA/BSc Sport and Exercise Studies and Zoology

Duration: 3FT Hon

Entry Requirements: *Foundation:* Merit. *GCE:* 180-240. *IB:* 26. *BTEC NC:* DM. *BTEC ND:* MMP.

C601 BA/BSc Sports Development and Physical Activity & Health

Duration: 3FT Hon

Entry Requirements: Contact the institution for details.

C603 BSc Sports and Exercise Science

Duration: 3FT Hon

Entry Requirements: *GCE:* 200-240. *IB:* 26. *BTEC NC:* DM. *BTEC ND:* MMM.

006C HND Sport and Exercise Studies

Duration: 2FT HND

Entry Requirements: *GCE:* 60-80.

D52 DONCASTER COLLEGE

THE HUB
CHAPPELL DRIVE
SOUTH YORKSHIRE DN1 2RF

t: 01302 553610
e: he@don.ac.uk

// www.don.ac.uk

C600 BSc Sport, Exercise and Health Sciences (Top Up)

Duration: 1FT Hon

Entry Requirements: Contact the institution for details.

C601 FdSc Sport and Health Studies

Duration: 2FT Fdg

Entry Requirements: Contact the institution for details.

D86 DURHAM UNIVERSITY

DURHAM UNIVERSITY
UNIVERSITY OFFICE
DURHAM DH1 3HP

t: 0191 334 2000 f: 0191 334 6055
e: admissions@durham.ac.uk

// www.durham.ac.uk

C601 BA Sport

Duration: 3FT Hon

Entry Requirements: *GCE:* ABB. *SQAH:* BBBBC. *SQAAH:* BBC. *IB:* 34.

C602 BA Sport with Foundation

Duration: 4FT Hon

Entry Requirements: Interview required.

E25 EAST LANCASHIRE INSTITUTE OF HIGHER EDUCATION AT BLACKBURN COLLEGE

DUKE STREET
BLACKBURN BB2 1LH

t: 01254 292594 f: 01254 260749
e: he-admissions@blackburn.ac.uk

// www.elihe.ac.uk

CN62 FdA Exercise and Fitness Management

Duration: 2FT Fdg

Entry Requirements: *GCE:* 60-80.

CB69 FdSc Sports and Rehabilitation

Duration: 2FT Fdg

Entry Requirements: Contact the institution for details.

C601 FdA Sports Development

Duration: 2FT Fdg

Entry Requirements: Contact the institution for details.

E28 UNIVERSITY OF EAST LONDON

DOCKLANDS CAMPUS
UNIVERSITY WAY
LONDON E16 2RD

t: 020 8223 2835 f: 020 8223 2978
e: admiss@uel.ac.uk

// www.uel.ac.uk

X3C6 BA Early Childhood Studies with Sports Development

Duration: 3FT Hon

Entry Requirements: *GCE:* 200. *IB:* 24. *BTEC NC:* DM. *BTEC ND:* MMP.

N5C6 BA Marketing with Sports Development

Duration: 3FT Hon

Entry Requirements: *GCE:* 200. *IB:* 24. *BTEC NC:* DM. *BTEC ND:* MMP.

W3C6 BA Music Culture with Sports Development

Duration: 3FT Hon

Entry Requirements: *GCE:* 200. *IB:* 24. *BTEC NC:* DM. *BTEC ND:* MMP. *OCR ND:* Merit. *OCR NED:* Pass.

B9C6 BSc Health Promotion with Sports Development

Duration: 3FT Hon

Entry Requirements: *GCE:* 200. *IB:* 24. *BTEC NC:* DM. *BTEC ND:* MMP.

C6N4 BSc Sports & Exercise Science with Accounting

Duration: 3FT Hon

Entry Requirements: *GCE:* 200. *IB:* 24. *BTEC NC:* DM. *BTEC ND:* MMP. *OCR ND:* Merit. *OCR NED:* Pass.

C6X9 BSc Sports & Exercise Science with Education & Community Development

Duration: 3FT Hon

Entry Requirements: *GCE:* 200. *IB:* 24. *BTEC NC:* DM. *BTEC ND:* MMP.

CG65 BSc Sports & Exercise Science/Information Technology

Duration: 3FT Hon

Entry Requirements: *GCE:* 200. *IB:* 24. *BTEC NC:* DM. *BTEC ND:* MMP.

B993 BSc Sports Development

Duration: 3FT Hon

Entry Requirements: *GCE:* 80.

C618 BSc Sports Development (Extended)

Duration: 4FT Hon

Entry Requirements: *GCE:* 80.

C6B1 BSc Sports Development with Human Biology

Duration: 3FT Hon

Entry Requirements: *GCE:* 200. *IB:* 24. *BTEC NC:* DM. *BTEC ND:* MMP. *OCR ND:* Merit. *OCR NED:* Pass.

C6BY BSc Sports Development with Public Health

Duration: 3FT Hon

Entry Requirements: *GCE:* 200. *IB:* 24. *BTEC NC:* DM. *BTEC ND:* MMP.

E42 EDGE HILL UNIVERSITY

ORMSKIRK
LANCASHIRE L39 4QP

t: 0800 195 5063 **f:** 01695 584355
e: enquiries@edgehill.ac.uk

// www.edgehill.ac.uk

C604 BA Sport Development

Duration: 3FT Deg

Entry Requirements: *GCE:* 240. *IB:* 28. *BTEC NC:* DD. *BTEC ND:* MMM. *OCR ND:* Distinction.

E59 EDINBURGH NAPIER UNIVERSITY

CRAIGLOCKHART CAMPUS
EDINBURGH EH14 1DJ

t: +44 (0)8452 60 60 40 **f:** 0131 455 6464
e: info@napier.ac.uk

// www.napier.ac.uk

C603 BSc Sport & Exercise Science (Sports Injuries top up)

Duration: 1FT Ord

Entry Requirements: HND required.

CB6X BSc Sport and Exercise Science (Sports Injuries)

Duration: 3FT/4FT Ord/Hon

Entry Requirements: *GCE:* 240.

E84 UNIVERSITY OF EXETER

LAVER BUILDING
NORTH PARK ROAD
EXETER
DEVON EX4 4QE

t: 01392 263855 **f:** 01392 263857/262479
e: admissions@exeter.ac.uk

// www.exeter.ac.uk/admissions

C602 BSc Exercise and Sport Sciences

Duration: 3FT Hon

Entry Requirements: *GCE:* AAB-BBB. *BTEC ND:* DDM.

G14 UNIVERSITY OF GLAMORGAN, CARDIFF AND PONTYPRIDD

ENQUIRIES AND ADMISSIONS UNIT
PONTYPRIDD CF37 1DL

t: 0800 716925 **f:** 01443 654050
e: enquiries@glam.ac.uk

// www.glam.ac.uk

C604 BSc Sports Studies

Duration: 3FT Hon

Entry Requirements: *GCE:* 240.

G42 GLASGOW CALEDONIAN UNIVERSITY

CITY CAMPUS
COWCADDENS ROAD
GLASGOW G4 0BA

t: 0141 331 3000 **f:** 0141 331 3449
e: admissions@gcal.ac.uk

// www.gcal.ac.uk

CN65 BA Sport and Active Lifestyles Promotion

Duration: 4FT Hon

Entry Requirements: *GCE:* CC.

G50 THE UNIVERSITY OF GLOUCESTERSHIRE

HARDWICK CAMPUS
ST PAUL'S ROAD
CHELTENHAM GL50 4BS

t: 01242 714501 **f:** 01242 543334
e: admissions@glos.ac.uk

// www.glos.ac.uk

CL65 BA/BSc Sports Development and Integrated Youth Practice

Duration: 3FT Hon

Entry Requirements: *GCE:* 200-300.

C605 BSc Applied Sport & Exercise Studies

Duration: 1FT Hon

Entry Requirements: HND required.

C601 BSc Sports Development

Duration: 3FT Hon

Entry Requirements: *GCE:* 240-300.

C607 FdSc Sports (Development)

Duration: 2FT Fdg

Entry Requirements: *GCE:* 80-100. Interview required.

G53 GLYNDWR UNIVERSITY
PLAS COCH
MOLD ROAD
WREXHAM LL11 2AW
t: 01978 293439 f: 01978 290008
e: SID@glyndwr.ac.uk
// www.glyndwr.ac.uk

C613 BA Community Sport Development
Duration: 3FT Hon

Entry Requirements: *GCE:* 200.

G70 UNIVERSITY OF GREENWICH
GREENWICH CAMPUS
OLD ROYAL NAVAL COLLEGE
PARK ROW
LONDON SE10 9LS
t: 0800 005 006 f: 020 8331 8145
e: courseinfo@gre.ac.uk
// www.gre.ac.uk

C603 BA Community Sport
Duration: 3FT Hon

Entry Requirements: Contact the institution for details.

C605 FdSc Sports Studies
Duration: 2FT Fdg

Entry Requirements: *GCE:* 100. *IB:* 24.

CL65 FdA Sports Studies (Community Sports Development)
Duration: 2FT Fdg

Entry Requirements: Contact the institution for details.

H36 UNIVERSITY OF HERTFORDSHIRE
UNIVERSITY ADMISSIONS SERVICE
COLLEGE LANE
HATFIELD
HERTS AL10 9AB
t: 01707 284800 f: 01707 284870
// www.herts.ac.uk

N1C6 BSc Business/Sports Studies
Duration: 3FT/4SW Hon

Entry Requirements: *GCE:* 260.

G4C6 BSc Computing/Sports Studies
Duration: 3FT/4SW Hon

Entry Requirements: *GCE:* 260.

H6C6 BSc Digital Media Technology/Sports Studies
Duration: 3FT/4SW Hon

Entry Requirements: *GCE:* 260.

RC86 BSc European Studies/Sports Studies
Duration: 3FT/4SW Hon

Entry Requirements: Contact the institution for details.

B1C6 BSc Human Biology/Sports Studies
Duration: 3FT/4SW Hon

Entry Requirements: Contact the institution for details.

L7C6 BSc Human Geography/Sports Studies
Duration: 3FT/4SW Hon

Entry Requirements: *GCE:* 260.

G2C6 BSc Management Science/Sports Studies
Duration: 3FT/4SW Hon

Entry Requirements: Contact the institution for details.

C8C6 BSc Psychology/Sports Studies
Duration: 3FT/4SW Hon

Entry Requirements: *GCE:* 260.

C602 BSc Sports Studies
Duration: 3FT/4SW Hon

Entry Requirements: *GCE:* 260.

C6R1 BSc Sports Studies/French
Duration: 3FT/4SW Hon

Entry Requirements: *GCE:* 220.

C6B9 BSc Sports Studies/Health Studies
Duration: 3FT/4SW Hon

Entry Requirements: Contact the institution for details.

C6L7 BSc Sports Studies/Human Geography
Duration: 3FT/4SW Hon

Entry Requirements: *GCE:* 260.

C6C8 BSc Sports Studies/Psychology
Duration: 3FT/4SW Hon

Entry Requirements: *GCE:* 260.

C601 FdSc Sports Studies
Duration: 2FT Fdg

Entry Requirements: *GCE:* 260.

H49 UHI MILLENNIUM INSTITUTE

UHI EXECUTIVE OFFICE
NESS WALK
INVERNESS
SCOTLAND IV3 5SQ

t: 01463 279000 f: 01463 279001
e: info@uhi.ac.uk
// www.uhi.ac.uk

206C HNC Fitness, Health & Exercise
Duration: 1FT HNC

Entry Requirements: *SQAH:* C.

H54 HOPWOOD HALL COLLEGE

ST MARY'S GATE
ROCHDALE
LANCS OL12 6RY

t: 01706 345346 f: 01706 641426
e: enquiries@hopwood.ac.uk
// www.hopwood.ac.uk

C600 FdSc Sports Development
Duration: 2FT Fdg

Entry Requirements: Contact the institution for details.

H60 THE UNIVERSITY OF HUDDERSFIELD

QUEENSGATE
HUDDERSFIELD HD1 3DH

t: 01484 473969 f: 01484 472765
e: admissionsandrecords@hud.ac.uk
// www.hud.ac.uk

C6B9 BSc Exercise, Physical Activity and Health
Duration: 3FT Hon

Entry Requirements: *GCE:* 220-240. *SQAH:* BBBB. *IB:* 26.

H73 HULL COLLEGE

QUEEN'S GARDENS
HULL HU1 3DG

t: 01482 329943 f: 01482 598733
e: info@hull-college.ac.uk
// www.hull-college.ac.uk

C600 FdA Sports Studies
Duration: 2FT Fdg

Entry Requirements: Contact the institution for details.

K24 THE UNIVERSITY OF KENT

INFORMATION, RECRUITMENT & ADMISSIONS
REGISTRY
UNIVERSITY OF KENT
CANTERBURY. KENT CT2 7NZ

t: 01227 827272 f: 01227 827077
e: information@kent.ac.uk
// www.kent.ac.uk

C601 BA Sport and Exercise Management
Duration: 3FT Hon

Entry Requirements: *GCE:* 240. *SQAH:* ABBCC. *IB:* 27. *BTEC NC:* DD. *BTEC ND:* MMM. *OCR ND:* Distinction.

K84 KINGSTON UNIVERSITY

STUDENT INFORMATION & ADVICE CENTRE
COOPER HOUSE
40-46 SURBITON ROAD
KINGSTON UPON THAMES KT1 2HX

t: 020 8547 7053 f: 020 8547 7080
e: aps@kingston.ac.uk
// www.kingston.ac.uk

CB64 BSc Exercise, Nutrition and Health Foundation Year
Duration: 4FT/5SW Hon

Entry Requirements: *GCE:* 260.

BC4P BSc Nutrition and Sport Science
Duration: 3FT Hon

Entry Requirements: *GCE:* 200-280.

K90 KIRKLEES COLLEGE

HALIFAX ROAD
DEWSBURY
WEST YORKSHIRE WF13 2AS

t: 01924 436221 f: 01924 457047

BC96 FdSc Health Related Exercise & Fitness
Duration: 2FT Fdg

Entry Requirements: Contact the institution for details.

L05 LAKES COLLEGE - WEST CUMBRIA

HALLWOOD ROAD
LILLYHALL
WORKINGTON CA14 4JN

t: 01946 839300 f: 01946 839302
e: student.services@lcwc.ac.uk
// www.lakescollegewestcumbria.ac.uk

CB69 FdSc Physical Activity & Health
Duration: 2FT Fdg

Entry Requirements: Contact the institution for details.

L24 LEEDS TRINITY & ALL SAINTS (ACCREDITED COLLEGE OF THE UNIVERSITY OF LEEDS)

BROWNBERRIE LANE
HORSFORTH
LEEDS LS18 5HD

t: 0113 283 7150 f: 0113 283 7222
e: enquiries@leedstrinity.ac.uk
// www.leedstrinity.ac.uk

CN6M BA Sports Development and Marketing
Duration: 3FT Hon

Entry Requirements: GCE: 240. IB: 24. BTEC NC: PP. BTEC ND: PPP.

CX63 BA Sports Development and PE
Duration: 3FT Hon

Entry Requirements: GCE: 240. IB: 24. BTEC NC: PP. BTEC ND: PPP.

C6C8 BSc Sport & Exercise with Psychology
Duration: 3FT Hon

Entry Requirements: GCE: 240. IB: 24. BTEC NC: PP. BTEC ND: PPP.

CB64 BSc Sport, Health, Exercise and Nutrition
Duration: 3FT Hon

Entry Requirements: GCE: 240. IB: 24. BTEC NC: PP. BTEC ND: PPP.

L27 LEEDS METROPOLITAN UNIVERSITY

COURSE ENQUIRIES OFFICE
CIVIC QUARTER
LEEDS LS1 3HE

t: 0113 81 23113 f: 0113 81 23129
e: course-enquiries@leedsmet.ac.uk
// www.leedsmet.ac.uk

CN6G BA Sport, Leisure & Culture
Duration: 3FT Hon

Entry Requirements: GCE: 240. BTEC NC: DD. BTEC ND: MMM. OCR ND: Distinction.

CB6X BSc Sports & Exercise Therapy
Duration: 3FT Hon

Entry Requirements: GCE: 260.

C605 BSc Sports Performance
Duration: 1FT Hon

Entry Requirements: Contact the institution for details.

CW62 BSc Sports Performance and Digital Media
Duration: 3FT/4SW Hon

Entry Requirements: GCE: 160. IB: 24.

CN68 BSc Sports Performance and Events Management
Duration: 3FT/4SW Hon

Entry Requirements: Contact the institution for details.

L39 UNIVERSITY OF LINCOLN

ADMISSIONS
BRAYFORD POOL
LINCOLN LN6 7TS

t: 01522 886097 f: 01522 886146
e: admissions@lincoln.ac.uk
// www.lincoln.ac.uk

C604 BSc Golf Science and Development
Duration: 3FT Hon

Entry Requirements: GCE: 240.

L42 LINCOLN COLLEGE

MONKS ROAD
LINCOLN LN2 5HQ

t: 01522 876000 f: 01522 876200
e: enquiries@lincolncollege.ac.uk
// www.lincolncollege.ac.uk

CB69 FdSc Sport Performance and Exercise Development
Duration: 2FT Hon

Entry Requirements: Contact the institution for details.

L46 LIVERPOOL HOPE UNIVERSITY

HOPE PARK
LIVERPOOL L16 9JD

t: 0151 291 3295 f: 0151 291 2050
e: admission@hope.ac.uk
// www.hope.ac.uk

LCH6 BA Applied Social Science and Football Studies
Duration: 3FT Hon

Entry Requirements: GCE: 240. IB: 25.

CN61 BA Business and Sports Development
Duration: 3FT Hon

Entry Requirements: GCE: 240. IB: 25.

WC56 BA Dance and Football Studies
Duration: 3FT Hon

Entry Requirements: GCE: 240. IB: 25. Interview required.

XC16 BA Disability Studies and Football Studies
Duration: 3FT Hon

Entry Requirements: GCE: 240. IB: 25.

CX61 BA Disability Studies and Sport Studies
Duration: 3FT Hon

Entry Requirements: *GCE:* 240. *IB:* 25.

CX6D BA Disability Studies and Sports Development
Duration: 3FT Hon

Entry Requirements: *GCE:* 240. *IB:* 25.

WC46 BA Drama & Theatre Studies and Sport Studies
Duration: 3FT Hon

Entry Requirements: *GCE:* 240. *IB:* 25.

XC36 BA Early Childhood Studies and Football Studies
Duration: 3FT Hon

Entry Requirements: *GCE:* 240. *IB:* 25.

CXP3 BA Education Studies and Sports Development
Duration: 3FT Hon

Entry Requirements: *GCE:* 240. *IB:* 25.

QC3P BA English Language and Football Studies
Duration: 3FT Hon

Entry Requirements: *GCE:* 240. *IB:* 25.

QC3Q BA English Literature and Football Studies
Duration: 3FT Hon

Entry Requirements: *GCE:* 240. *IB:* 25.

CQ6J BA English Literature and Sports Development
Duration: 3FT Hon

Entry Requirements: *GCE:* 240. *IB:* 25.

WC16 BA Fine Art and Football Studies
Duration: 3FT Hon

Entry Requirements: *GCE:* 240. *IB:* 25.

WC1Q BA Fine Art and Sport Studies
Duration: 3FT Hon

Entry Requirements: *GCE:* 240. *IB:* 25.

WCC6 BA Fine Art and Sports Development
Duration: 3FT Hon

Entry Requirements: *GCE:* 240. *IB:* 25.

CV6C BA Football Studies and History
Duration: 3FT Hon

Entry Requirements: *GCE:* 240. *IB:* 25.

CX6H BA Football Studies and Inclusive Education
Duration: 3FT Hon

Entry Requirements: *GCE:* 240. *IB:* 25.

CL6F BA Football Studies and International Studies
Duration: 3FT Hon

Entry Requirements: *GCE:* 240. *IB:* 25.

CM6C BA Football Studies and Law
Duration: 3FT Hon

Entry Requirements: *GCE:* 240. *IB:* 25.

CN65 BA Football Studies and Marketing
Duration: 3FT Hon

Entry Requirements: *GCE:* 240. *IB:* 25.

CW6H BA Football Studies and Music
Duration: 3FT Hon

Entry Requirements: *GCE:* 240. *IB:* 25.

CV66 BA Football Studies and Theology & Religious Studies
Duration: 3FT Hon

Entry Requirements: *GCE:* 240. *IB:* 25.

CN6V BA Football Studies and Tourism
Duration: 3FT Hon

Entry Requirements: *GCE:* 240. *IB:* 25.

VC16 BA History and Sport Studies
Duration: 3FT Hon

Entry Requirements: *GCE:* 240. *IB:* 25.

CM61 BA Law and Sports Development
Duration: 3FT Hon

Entry Requirements: *GCE:* 240. *IB:* 25.

NC56 BA Marketing and Sport Studies
Duration: 3FT Hon

Entry Requirements: *GCE:* 240. *IB:* 25.

CN6M BA Marketing and Sports Development
Duration: 3FT Hon

Entry Requirements: *GCE:* 240. *IB:* 25.

VC56 BA Philosophy & Ethics and Sports Development
Duration: 3FT Hon

Entry Requirements: *GCE:* 240. *IB:* 25.

LC2Q BA Politics and Sport Studies
Duration: 3FT Hon

Entry Requirements: *GCE:* 240. *IB:* 25.

CL62 BA Politics and Sports Development
Duration: 3FT Hon

Entry Requirements: *GCE:* 240. *IB:* 25.

X1CP BA Primary Teaching with Sport Studies
Duration: 4FT Hon

Entry Requirements: *GCE:* 280. *IB:* 25. Interview required.

GC46 BSc Computing and Football Studies
Duration: 3FT Hon

Entry Requirements: *GCE:* 240. *IB:* 25.

CC16 BSc Environmental Biology and Football Studies
Duration: 3FT Hon

Entry Requirements: *GCE:* 240. *IB:* 25.

CF68 BSc Football Studies and Geography
Duration: 3FT Hon

Entry Requirements: *GCE:* 240. *IB:* 25.

CB6X BSc Football Studies and Health
Duration: 3FT Hon

Entry Requirements: *GCE:* 240. *IB:* 25.

CB6C BSc Football Studies and Human Biology
Duration: 3FT Hon

Entry Requirements: *GCE:* 240. *IB:* 25.

CG6M BSc Football Studies and Information Technology
Duration: 3FT Hon

Entry Requirements: *GCE:* 240. *IB:* 25.

CB64 BSc Football Studies and Nutrition
Duration: 3FT Hon

Entry Requirements: *GCE:* 240. *IB:* 25.

CN68 BSc Football Studies and Outdoor Recreation
Duration: 3FT Hon

Entry Requirements: *GCE:* 240. *IB:* 25.

C602 BSc Football Studies and Sport Development
Duration: 3FT Hon

Entry Requirements: *GCE:* 240. *IB:* 25.

C603 BSc Football Studies and Sport Studies
Duration: 3FT Hon

Entry Requirements: *GCE:* 240. *IB:* 25.

FC86 BSc Geography and Sport Studies
Duration: 3FT Hon

Entry Requirements: *GCE:* 240. *IB:* 25.

CBP9 BSc Health and Sport Studies
Duration: 3FT Hon

Entry Requirements: *GCE:* 240. *IB:* 25.

CB61 BSc Human Biology and Sport Studies
Duration: 3FT Hon

Entry Requirements: *GCE:* 240. *IB:* 25.

NC86 BSc Outdoor Recreation and Sport Studies
Duration: 3FT Hon

Entry Requirements: *GCE:* 240. *IB:* 25.

BCXP BSc Sport & Health Studies
Duration: 3FT Hon

Entry Requirements: *GCE:* 240. *IB:* 25.

L51 LIVERPOOL JOHN MOORES UNIVERSITY
ROSCOE COURT
4 RODNEY STREET
LIVERPOOL L1 2TZ
t: 0151 231 5090 f: 0151 231 3462
e: recruitment@ljmu.ac.uk
// www.ljmu.ac.uk

C601 BSc Exercise Science
Duration: 3FT Hon

Entry Requirements: *GCE:* 40-100.

C6J9 BSc Sports Technology

Duration: 3FT/4SW Hon

Entry Requirements: *GCE:* 240-280. *IB:* 27. *BTEC NC:* DD. *BTEC ND:* MMM.

L68 LONDON METROPOLITAN UNIVERSITY

166-220 HOLLOWAY ROAD
LONDON N7 8DB

t: 020 7133 4200
e: admissions@londonmet.ac.uk

// www.londonmet.ac.uk

C600 BSc Sports Product Design

Duration: 3FT/4SW Hon

Entry Requirements: *GCE:* 200. *IB:* 28.

CX6C FdA Community Sport Coaching & Management

Duration: 2FT Fdg

Entry Requirements: *GCE:* 100. *IB:* 28.

L75 LONDON SOUTH BANK UNIVERSITY

103 BOROUGH ROAD
LONDON SE1 0AA

t: 020 7815 7815 f: 020 7815 8273
e: enquiry@lsbu.ac.uk

// www.lsbu.ac.uk

H7C6 BSc Sports Product Design

Duration: 3FT/4SW Hon

Entry Requirements: *GCE:* 160. *IB:* 24. *BTEC NC:* MM. *BTEC ND:* MPP.

L79 LOUGHBOROUGH UNIVERSITY

LOUGHBOROUGH
LEICESTERSHIRE LE11 3TU

t: 01509 223522 f: 01509 223905
e: admissions@lboro.ac.uk

// www.lboro.ac.uk

CH67 BSc Sports Technology

Duration: 3FT Hon

Entry Requirements: *GCE:* 320. *IB:* 33.

M40 THE MANCHESTER METROPOLITAN UNIVERSITY

ADMISSIONS OFFICE
ALL SAINTS (GMS)
ALL SAINTS
MANCHESTER M15 6BH

t: 0161 247 2000

// www.mmu.ac.uk

LCN6 BA Abuse Studies/Sport Development

Duration: 3FT Hon

Entry Requirements: *BTEC ND:* MMM.

LC56 BA Childhood & Youth Studies/Exercise & Physical Activity

Duration: 3FT Hon

Entry Requirements: *BTEC ND:* MMM.

LC5P BA Childhood & Youth Studies/Sport Development

Duration: 3FT Hon

Entry Requirements: *BTEC ND:* MMM.

XC1Q BA Coaching Studies/Sport Development

Duration: 3FT Hon

Entry Requirements: Contact the institution for details.

WCHP BA Creative Music Production/Sport Development

Duration: 3FT Hon

Entry Requirements: Contact the institution for details.

LCHP BA Crime Studies/Sport Development

Duration: 3FT Hon

Entry Requirements: Contact the institution for details.

LC66 BA Cultural Studies/Exercise & Physical Activity

Duration: 3FT Hon

Entry Requirements: *GCE:* 260. *BTEC ND:* MMM.

WCK6 BA Drama/Outdoor Studies

Duration: 3FT Hon

Entry Requirements: *GCE:* 260. *BTEC ND:* DMM.

XCH6 BA Education Studies/Exercise & Physical Activity

Duration: 3FT Hon

Entry Requirements: *GCE:* 260. *BTEC ND:* MMM.

CBQ9 BA Exercise & Physical Activity/Health Studies

Duration: 3FT Hon

Entry Requirements: *GCE:* 260. *BTEC ND:* MMM.

CM69 BA Exercise & Physical Activity/Legal Studies

Duration: 3FT Hon

Entry Requirements: *GCE:* 260. *BTEC ND:* MMM.

CVP5 BA Exercise & Physical Activity/Philosophy

Duration: 3FT Hon

Entry Requirements: *GCE:* 260. *BTEC ND:* MMM.

WCJ6 BA Exercise & Physical Activity/Popular Music

Duration: 3FT Hon

Entry Requirements: *GCE:* 260. *BTEC ND:* DMM.

NCM6 BA Marketing/Sport Development

Duration: 3FT Hon

Entry Requirements: *GCE:* 260. *BTEC ND:* MMM.

WCJP BA Music/Sport Development

Duration: 3FT Hon

Entry Requirements: Contact the institution for details.

CV65 BA Philosophy/Sport

Duration: 3FT Hon

Entry Requirements: *GCE:* 260. *IB:* 28. *BTEC ND:* MMM.

LCHQ BA Sociology/Sport Development

Duration: 3FT Hon

Entry Requirements: *GCE:* 260. *BTEC ND:* MMM.

CXP3 BA/BSc Childhood & Youth Studies/Sport

Duration: 3FT Hon

Entry Requirements: *GCE:* 260. *IB:* 28. *BTEC ND:* MMM.

WC3P BA/BSc Creative Music Production/Exercise & Physical Activity

Duration: 3FT Hon

Entry Requirements: Contact the institution for details.

WC3Q BA/BSc Creative Music Production/Outdoor Studies

Duration: 3FT Hon

Entry Requirements: Contact the institution for details.

JC96 BA/BSc Creative Music Production/Sport

Duration: 3FT Hon

Entry Requirements: Contact the institution for details.

QC36 BA/BSc English/Outdoor Studies

Duration: 3FT Hon

Entry Requirements: *GCE:* 260. *BTEC ND:* MMM.

GC5P BA/BSc IT Management/Exercise & Physical Activity

Duration: 3FT Hon

Entry Requirements: HND required.

GCM6 BA/BSc IT Management/Sport

Duration: 3FT Hon

Entry Requirements: Contact the institution for details.

LC96 BA/BSc Justice and the Environment/Exercise & Physical Activity

Duration: 3FT Hon

Entry Requirements: Contact the institution for details.

LC9Q BA/BSc Justice and the Environment/Outdoor Studies

Duration: 3FT Hon

Entry Requirements: Contact the institution for details.

NC56 BA/BSc Marketing/Outdoor Studies

Duration: 3FT Hon

Entry Requirements: *GCE:* 260. *BTEC ND:* MMM.

WCHQ BA/BSc Music/Outdoor Studies

Duration: 3FT Hon

Entry Requirements: Contact the institution for details.

CL6H BA/BSc Outdoor Studies/Crime Studies

Duration: 3FT Hon

Entry Requirements: *GCE:* 40.

CV6M BA/BSc Outdoor Studies/Philosophy

Duration: 3FT Hon

Entry Requirements: *GCE:* 260. *BTEC ND:* MMM.

CW6H BA/BSc Popular Music/Sport

Duration: 3FT Hon

Entry Requirements: *GCE:* 260. *BTEC ND:* DMM.

CF68 BSc Exercise & Physical Activity/Geography

Duration: 3FT Hon

Entry Requirements: *GCE:* 260. *BTEC ND:* MMM.

C605 BSc Exercise & Physical Activity/Outdoor Studies

Duration: 3FT Hon

Entry Requirements: *GCE:* 260. *BTEC ND:* MMM.

CCP8 BSc Exercise & Physical Activity/Psychology

Duration: 3FT Hon

Entry Requirements: *GCE:* 260. *BTEC ND:* MMM.

C606 BSc Exercise & Physical Activity/Sport Development

Duration: 3FT Hon

Entry Requirements: *GCE:* 260. *BTEC ND:* MMM.

C601 BSc Outdoor Studies

Duration: 3FT Hon

Entry Requirements: *GCE:* 200. *SQAH:* BBBCC.

C607 BSc Sport/Sport Development

Duration: 3FT Hon

Entry Requirements: *GCE:* 260. *BTEC ND:* MMM.

M80 MIDDLESEX UNIVERSITY

MIDDLESEX UNIVERSITY
THE BURROUGHS
LONDON NW4 4BT

t: 020 8411 5555 f: 020 8411 5649
e: enquiries@mdx.ac.uk

// www.mdx.ac.uk

C605 FdSc Health and Fitness

Duration: 2FT Fdg

Entry Requirements: Contact the institution for details.

N23 NEWCASTLE COLLEGE

STUDENT SERVICES
RYE HILL CAMPUS
SCOTSWOOD ROAD
NEWCASTLE UPON TYNE NE4 7SA

t: 0191 200 4000 f: 0191 200 4349
e: enquiries@ncl-coll.ac.uk

// www.newcastlecollege.co.uk

BC96 BSc Applied Health & Exercise Science (Top-up)

Duration: 1FT Hon

Entry Requirements: HND required.

C606 FdSc Applied Health and Exercise Science

Duration: 2FT Fdg

Entry Requirements: *GCE:* 80-120. *BTEC NC:* PP. *BTEC ND:* PPP.

CN62 FdA Applied Sport Management and Development

Duration: 2FT Fdg

Entry Requirements: *GCE:* 80-120. *BTEC NC:* PP. *BTEC ND:* PPP.

N28 NEW COLLEGE DURHAM

FRAMWELLGATE MOOR CENTRE
DURHAM DH1 5ES

t: 0191 375 4210/4211 f: 0191 375 4222
e: admissions@newdur.ac.uk

// www.newdur.ac.uk

C600 FdSc Sport and Exercise Studies

Duration: 2FT Fdg

Entry Requirements: *GCE:* 40. *BTEC NC:* PP. *BTEC ND:* PPP.

N36 NEWMAN UNIVERSITY COLLEGE, BIRMINGHAM

GENNERS LANE
BARTLEY GREEN
BIRMINGHAM B32 3NT

t: 0121 476 1181 f: 0121 476 1196
e: registry@newman.ac.uk

// www.newman.ac.uk

XX13 BA Sports Studies and Education Studies

Duration: 3FT Hon

Entry Requirements: *GCE:* 180-240. *IB:* 24. *BTEC NC:* MM. *BTEC ND:* MMP.

C6W1 BA Sports Studies with Art & Design

Duration: 3FT Hon

Entry Requirements: *GCE:* 180-240. *IB:* 24. *BTEC NC:* MM. *BTEC ND:* MMP.

C6B9 BA Sports Studies with Counselling

Duration: 3FT Hon

Entry Requirements: *GCE:* 180-240. *IB:* 24. *BTEC NC:* MM. *BTEC ND:* MMP.

C6W8 BA Sports Studies with Creative Writing

Duration: 3FT Hon

Entry Requirements: *GCE:* 180-240. *IB:* 24. *BTEC NC:* MM. *BTEC ND:* MMP.

C6V5 BA Sports Studies with Philosophy & Theology
Duration: 3FT Hon

Entry Requirements: *GCE:* 180-240. *IB:* 24. *BTEC NC:* MM. *BTEC ND:* MMP.

LC56 BA Working with Children Young People & Families and Sports Studies
Duration: 3FT Hon

Entry Requirements: *GCE:* 180-240. *IB:* 24. *BTEC NC:* MM. *BTEC ND:* MMP.

GC56 BSc IT and Sports Studies
Duration: 3FT Hon

Entry Requirements: *GCE:* 180-240. *IB:* 24. *BTEC NC:* MM. *BTEC ND:* MMP.

G5C6 BSc IT with Sport Studies
Duration: 3FT Hon

Entry Requirements: *GCE:* 180-240. *IB:* 24. *BTEC NC:* MM. *BTEC ND:* MMP.

C600 BSc Sports Studies
Duration: 3FT Hon

Entry Requirements: *GCE:* 200-240. *IB:* 24. *BTEC NC:* DM. *BTEC ND:* MMM.

C6G5 BSc Sports Studies with IT
Duration: 3FT Hon

Entry Requirements: *GCE:* 180-240. *IB:* 24. *BTEC NC:* MM. *BTEC ND:* MMP.

C6C8 BSc Sports Studies with Social & Applied Psychology
Duration: 3FT Hon

Entry Requirements: *GCE:* 180-240. *IB:* 24. *BTEC NC:* MM. *BTEC ND:* MMP.

N37 UNIVERSITY OF WALES, NEWPORT
CAERLEON CAMPUS
PO BOX 101
NEWPORT
SOUTH WALES NP18 3YH
t: 01633 432030 f: 01633 432850
e: admissions@newport.ac.uk
// www.newport.ac.uk

CM62 BA/BSc Sport and Youth Justice
Duration: 3FT Hon

Entry Requirements: *GCE:* 200-240. *IB:* 24. Interview required.

C600 BSc Sports Studies
Duration: 3FT Hon

Entry Requirements: *GCE:* 280. *IB:* 24. Interview required.

N38 UNIVERSITY OF NORTHAMPTON
PARK CAMPUS
BOUGHTON GREEN ROAD
NORTHAMPTON NN2 7AL
t: 0800 358 2232 f: 01604 722083
e: admissions@northampton.ac.uk
// www.northampton.ac.uk

T7CP BA American Literature & Film/Sport Studies
Duration: 3FT Hon

Entry Requirements: *GCE:* 220-260. *SQAH:* AAB-DDDD. *IB:* 24.

T7C6 BA American Studies/Sport Studies
Duration: 3FT Hon

Entry Requirements: *GCE:* 220-260. *SQAH:* AAB-BBBB. *IB:* 24.

N1CP BA Business Entrepreneurship/Sport Studies
Duration: 3FT Hon

Entry Requirements: *GCE:* 220-260. *SQAH:* AAB-BBBB. *IB:* 24.

N1C6 BA Business/Sport Studies
Duration: 3FT Hon

Entry Requirements: *GCE:* 220-260. *SQAH:* AAB-BBBB. *IB:* 24.

W8C6 BA Creative Writing/Sport Studies
Duration: 3FT Hon

Entry Requirements: *GCE:* 220-260. *SQAH:* AAB-BBBB. *IB:* 24.

M9C6 BA Criminology/Sport Studies
Duration: 3FT Hon

Entry Requirements: *GCE:* 220-260. *SQAH:* AAB-BBBB. *IB:* 24.

QC36 BA English Language/Sport Studies
Duration: 3FT Hon

Entry Requirements: *GCE:* 220-260. *SQAH:* AAB-BBBB. *IB:* 24.

W1C6 BA Fine Art Painting & Drawing/Sport Studies
Duration: 3FT Hon

Entry Requirements: *GCE:* 220-260. *SQAH:* AAB-BBBB. *IB:* 24.

R1C6 BA French/Sport Studies
Duration: 3FT Hon

Entry Requirements: *GCE:* 220-260. *SQAH:* AAB-BBBB. *IB:* 24.

V1C6 BA History/Sport Studies
Duration: 3FT Hon
Entry Requirements: *GCE:* 220-260. *SQAH:* AAB-BBBB. *IB:* 24.

L7C6 BA Human Geography/Sport Studies
Duration: 3FT Hon
Entry Requirements: *GCE:* 220-260. *SQAH:* AAB-BBBB. *IB:* 24.

N6C6 BA Human Resource Management/Sport Studies
Duration: 3FT Hon
Entry Requirements: *GCE:* 220-260. *SQAH:* AAB-BBBB. *IB:* 24.

P4C6 BA Magazine Publishing/Sport Studies
Duration: 3FT Hon
Entry Requirements: *GCE:* 220-260. *SQAH:* AAB-BBBB. *IB:* 24.

W3C6 BA Popular Music/Sport Studies
Duration: 3FT Hon
Entry Requirements: *GCE:* 220-260. *SQAH:* AAB-BBBB. *IB:* 24.

L3C6 BA Sociology/Sport Studies
Duration: 3FT Hon
Entry Requirements: *GCE:* 220-260. *SQAH:* AAB-BBBB. *IB:* 24.

C602 BA Sport Development
Duration: 3FT Hon
Entry Requirements: *GCE:* 220-260. *SQAH:* AAB-BBBB. *IB:* 24.

C604 BA Sport Development (2 year fast track)
Duration: 2FT Hon
Entry Requirements: *GCE:* 220-260. *SQAH:* AAB-BBBB. *IB:* 24.

C6TR BA Sport Studies/American Literature & Film
Duration: 3FT Hon
Entry Requirements: *GCE:* 220-260. *SQAH:* AAB-BBBB. *IB:* 24.

C6NF BA Sport Studies/Business Entrepreneurship
Duration: 3FT Hon
Entry Requirements: *GCE:* 220-260. *SQAH:* AAB-BBBB. *IB:* 24.

C6W5 BA Sport Studies/Dance
Duration: 3FT Hon
Entry Requirements: *GCE:* 220-260. *SQAH:* AAB-BBBB. *IB:* 24.

C6X3 BA Sport Studies/Education Studies
Duration: 3FT Hon
Entry Requirements: *GCE:* 220-260. *SQAH:* AAB-BBBB. *IB:* 24.

C6Q3 BA Sport Studies/English Language
Duration: 3FT Hon
Entry Requirements: *GCE:* 200.

C6W6 BA Sport Studies/Film & Television Studies
Duration: 3FT Hon
Entry Requirements: *GCE:* 220-260. *SQAH:* AAB-BBBB. *IB:* 24.

C6W1 BA Sport Studies/Fine Art Painting & Drawing
Duration: 3FT Hon
Entry Requirements: *GCE:* 220-260. *SQAH:* AAB-BBBB. *IB:* 24.

C6L7 BA Sport Studies/Human Geography
Duration: 3FT Hon
Entry Requirements: *GCE:* 220-260. *SQAH:* AAB-BBBB. *IB:* 24.

C6N6 BA Sport Studies/Human Resource Management
Duration: 3FT Hon
Entry Requirements: *GCE:* 220-260. *SQAH:* AAB-BBBB. *IB:* 24.

C6N2 BA Sport Studies/Management
Duration: 3FT Hon
Entry Requirements: *GCE:* 220-260. *SQAH:* AAB-BBBB. *IB:* 24.

C6V5 BA Sport Studies/Philosophy
Duration: 3FT Hon
Entry Requirements: *GCE:* 220-260. *SQAH:* AAB-BBBB. *IB:* 24.

C6L2 BA Sport Studies/Politics
Duration: 3FT Hon
Entry Requirements: *GCE:* 220-260. *SQAH:* AAB-BBBB. *IB:* 24.

C6W3 BA Sport Studies/Popular Music
Duration: 3FT Hon
Entry Requirements: *GCE:* 220-260. *SQAH:* AAB-BBBB. *IB:* 24.

C6C8 BA Sport Studies/Psychology
Duration: 3FT Hon
Entry Requirements: *GCE:* 220-260. *SQAH:* AAB-BBBB. *IB:* 24.

C6N9 BA Sport Studies/Social Enterprise Development
Duration: 3FT Hon

Entry Requirements: *GCE:* 220-260. *SQAH:* AAB-BBBB. *IB:* 24.

C6L3 BA Sport Studies/Sociology
Duration: 3FT Hon

Entry Requirements: *GCE:* 220-260. *SQAH:* AAB-BBBB. *IB:* 24.

G5C6 BSc Business Computing Systems/Sport Studies
Duration: 3FT Hon

Entry Requirements: *GCE:* 220-260. *SQAH:* AAB-BBBB. *IB:* 24.

F8C6 BSc Physical Geography/Sport Studies
Duration: 3FT Hon

Entry Requirements: *GCE:* 220-260. *SQAH:* AAB-BBBB. *IB:* 24.

CC86 BSc Sport & Exercise Psychology
Duration: 3FT Hon

Entry Requirements: *GCE:* 220-260. *SQAH:* AAB-BBBB. *IB:* 24.

C600 BSc Sport & Exercise Science
Duration: 3FT Hon

Entry Requirements: *GCE:* 220-260. *SQAH:* AAB-BBBB. *IB:* 24.

C6D4 BSc Sport Studies with Equine Studies
Duration: 3FT Hon

Entry Requirements: *GCE:* 220-260. *SQAH:* AAB-BBBB. *IB:* 24.

C6FV BSc Sport Studies/Wastes Management
Duration: 3FT Hon

Entry Requirements: *GCE:* 220-260. *SQAH:* AAB-BBBB. *IB:* 24.

N82 NORWICH CITY COLLEGE OF FURTHER AND HIGHER EDUCATION (AN ASSOCIATE COLLEGE OF UEA)
IPSWICH ROAD
NORWICH
NORFOLK NR2 2LJ

t: 01603 773005 f: 01603 773301
e: admissions@ccn.ac.uk

// www.ccn.ac.uk

C600 FdA Sport, Health and Exercise
Duration: 2FT Fdg

Entry Requirements: Contact the institution for details.

N91 NOTTINGHAM TRENT UNIVERSITY
DRYDEN CENTRE
BURTON STREET
NOTTINGHAM NG1 4BU

t: +44 (0) 115 941 8418 f: +44 (0) 115 848 6063
e: admissions@ntu.ac.uk

// www.ntu.ac.uk/

CX63 BA Sport & Leisure and Educational Development
Duration: 3FT Hon

Entry Requirements: *GCE:* 200. *IB:* 28.

CN68 BSc Sport, Leisure and Outdoor Management
Duration: 3FT/4SW Hon

Entry Requirements: *GCE:* 240. *IB:* 26. *BTEC NC:* DD. *BTEC ND:* MMM.

O66 OXFORD BROOKES UNIVERSITY
ADMISSIONS OFFICE
HEADINGTON CAMPUS
GIPSY LANE
OXFORD OX3 0BP

t: 01865 483040 f: 01865 483983
e: admissions@brookes.ac.uk

// www.brookes.ac.uk

CY6A BA/BSc Exercise, Nutrition & Health/Combined Studies
Duration: 3FT Hon

Entry Requirements: *GCE:* BCC.

C605 BA/BSc Exercise, Nutrition & Health/Sports & Coaching Studies
Duration: 3FT Hon

Entry Requirements: *GCE:* BBC.

C603 BA/BSc Sport & Exercise Science/Sports & Coaching Studies
Duration: 3FT Hon

Entry Requirements: *GCE:* BBC.

DC46 BSc Environmental Management/Exercise, Nutrition and Health
Duration: 3FT Hon

Entry Requirements: *GCE:* BBC.

CCQ1 BSc Exercise, Nutrition & Health/Biology
Duration: 3FT Hon

Entry Requirements: *GCE:* BBC.

CC6D BSc Exercise, Nutrition & Health/Ecology

Duration: 3FT Hon

Entry Requirements: *GCE:* BBC.

CFPV BSc Exercise, Nutrition & Health/Environmental Sciences

Duration: 3FT Hon

Entry Requirements: *GCE:* BBC.

CB6C BSc Exercise, Nutrition & Health/Human Biology

Duration: 3FT Hon

Entry Requirements: *GCE:* BBC.

CB6L BSc Exercise, Nutrition & Health/Nutrition

Duration: 3FT Hon

Entry Requirements: *GCE:* BBC.

P60 UNIVERSITY OF PLYMOUTH
DRAKE CIRCUS
PLYMOUTH PL4 8AA
t: 01752 588037 **f:** 01752 588050
e: admissions@plymouth.ac.uk
// www.plymouth.ac.uk

C606 BSc Health and Fitness

Duration: 1FT Hon

Entry Requirements: HND required.

P63 UCP MARJON - UNIVERSITY COLLEGE PLYMOUTH ST MARK & ST JOHN
DERRIFORD ROAD
PLYMOUTH PL6 8BH
t: 01752 636890 **f:** 01752 636819
e: admissions@marjon.ac.uk
// www.ucpmarjon.ac.uk

L5CP BA Community Practice with Outdoor Adventure

Duration: 3FT Hon

Entry Requirements: *GCE:* 180.

C603 BA Outdoor Adventure with Sports Development

Duration: 3FT Hon

Entry Requirements: *GCE:* 180.

C601 BA Outdoor Studies

Duration: 1FT Hon

Entry Requirements: Contact the institution for details.

C602 BA Sports Development

Duration: 3FT Hon

Entry Requirements: *GCE:* 180.

C605 BA Sports Development with Outdoor Adventure

Duration: 3FT Hon

Entry Requirements: *GCE:* 180.

S03 THE UNIVERSITY OF SALFORD
SALFORD M5 4WT
t: 0161 295 4545 **f:** 0161 295 3126
e: ugadmissions-exrel@salford.ac.uk
// www.salford.ac.uk

CB69 BSc Exercise, Physical Activity and Health

Duration: 3FT Hon

Entry Requirements: *GCE:* 200. *IB:* 24. *BTEC NC:* DM. *BTEC ND:* MMP.

S18 THE UNIVERSITY OF SHEFFIELD
9 NORTHUMBERLAND ROAD
SHEFFIELD S10 2TT
t: 0114 222 1255 **f:** 0114 222 8032
e: ask@sheffield.ac.uk
// www.sheffield.ac.uk

CH63 MEng Sports Engineering

Duration: 4FT Hon

Entry Requirements: *GCE:* 340. *IB:* 32. Interview required.

S21 SHEFFIELD HALLAM UNIVERSITY
CITY CAMPUS
HOWARD STREET
SHEFFIELD S1 1WB
t: 0114 225 5555 **f:** 0114 225 2167
e: admissions@shu.ac.uk
// www.shu.ac.uk

CL65 BA Sport & Community Development

Duration: 3FT Hon

Entry Requirements: *GCE:* 200.

C6N2 BSc Sport Business Management

Duration: 3FT Hon

Entry Requirements: *GCE:* 200.

C6X3 BSc Sport Development with Coaching

Duration: 3FT Hon

Entry Requirements: *GCE:* 230.

C6G4 BSc Sport Technology

Duration: 3FT/4SW Hon

Entry Requirements: *GCE:* 220.

S27 UNIVERSITY OF SOUTHAMPTON

HIGHFIELD
SOUTHAMPTON SO17 1BJ

t: 023 8059 4732 f: 023 8059 3037
e: admissions@soton.ac.uk

// www.southampton.ac.uk

CN62 BA Managing and Developing Sport

Duration: 3FT Hon

Entry Requirements: *BTEC ND:* DDM.

S28 SOMERSET COLLEGE OF ARTS AND TECHNOLOGY

WELLINGTON ROAD
TAUNTON
SOMERSET TA1 5AX

t: 01823 366331 f: 01823 366418
e: enquiries@somerset.ac.uk

// www.somerset.ac.uk/student-
area/considering-a-degree.html

CN62 FdSc Sports Management and Development

Duration: 2FT Fdg

Entry Requirements: *GCE:* 80. *IB:* 24. *BTEC NC:* PP. *BTEC ND:* PPP.

S30 SOUTHAMPTON SOLENT UNIVERSITY

EAST PARK TERRACE
SOUTHAMPTON
HAMPSHIRE SO14 0RT

t: +44 (0) 23 8031 9039 f: + 44 (0)23 8022 2259
e: admissions@solent.ac.uk or ask@solent.ac.uk

// www.solent.ac.uk/

CN62 BA Football Studies

Duration: 3FT Hon

Entry Requirements: *GCE:* 240.

C6Q3 BA Football Studies with Language Fdn Year

Duration: 4FT Hon

Entry Requirements: Contact the institution for details.

CBP9 BA Health and Fitness Management

Duration: 3FT Hon

Entry Requirements: *GCE:* 220. *BTEC NC:* MM. *BTEC ND:* MPP.

LC56 BA Health Promotion and Fitness

Duration: 3FT Hon

Entry Requirements: *GCE:* 120.

C601 BA Sports Studies

Duration: 3FT Hon

Entry Requirements: *GCE:* 220.

C6ND BA Sports Studies with Business with Lang Fdn Year

Duration: 4FT Hon

Entry Requirements: Contact the institution for details.

BC96 BSc Health, Exercise and Physical Activity

Duration: 3FT Hon

Entry Requirements: *GCE:* 220.

S51 ST HELENS COLLEGE

WATER STREET
ST HELENS
MERSEYSIDE WA10 1PP

t: 01744 733766 f: 01744 623400
e: enquiries@sthelens.ac.uk

// www.sthelens.ac.uk

C610 FdSc Exercise, Health and Fitness

Duration: 2FT Fdg

Entry Requirements: *GCE:* 40. *IB:* 18. *BTEC NC:* PP. *BTEC ND:* PPP.

C6X9 FdSc Sports Development

Duration: 2FT Fdg

Entry Requirements: *GCE:* 40. *IB:* 18. *BTEC NC:* PP. *BTEC ND:* PPP.

S64 ST MARY'S UNIVERSITY COLLEGE, TWICKENHAM

WALDEGRAVE ROAD
STRAWBERRY HILL
MIDDLESEX TW1 4SX

t: 020 8240 4029 f: 020 8240 2361
e: admit@smuc.ac.uk

// www.smuc.ac.uk

BCY6 BSc Health & Exercise and Sport Science

Duration: 3FT Hon

Entry Requirements: *GCE:* 160-200. *BTEC NC:* MM. *BTEC ND:* MPP.

C607 BSc Strength and Conditioning

Duration: 3FT Hon

Entry Requirements: *GCE:* 180-200. *BTEC NC:* DM. *BTEC ND:* MMP.

Confused about courses?
Indecisive about institutions?
Stressed about student life?
Unsure about UCAS?
Frowning over finance?

Help is available.

Visit www.ucasbooks.com to view our range
of over 75 books covering all aspects
of entry into higher education.

www.ucasbooks.com

> Unlock your potential
It's as easy as 1, 2, 3.

1 **Search**

Use Course Search to look for courses in your subject;
find out about your chosen universities and colleges
and lots more.

2 **Apply**

Use our online system Apply to make your application to
higher education.

3 **Track**

Then use Track to monitor the progress of your application.

UCAS   helping students into higher education   **www.ucas.com**

CB6X FdA Sport, Health and Fitness

Duration: 2FT Fdg

Entry Requirements: *GCE:* 80-120.

S72 STAFFORDSHIRE UNIVERSITY

COLLEGE ROAD
STOKE ON TRENT ST4 2DE

t: 01782 292753 f: 01782 292740
e: admissions@staffs.ac.uk
// www.staffs.ac.uk

CN62 BA Sport and Leisure Management

Duration: 3FT Hon

Entry Requirements: *GCE:* 180-240. *IB:* 24. *BTEC NC:* DM. *BTEC ND:* MMM.

C602 BA Sports Studies

Duration: 3FT Hon

Entry Requirements: *GCE:* 180-240. *IB:* 24. *BTEC NC:* DM. *BTEC ND:* MMM.

C600 BSc Sports Studies

Duration: 3FT Hon

Entry Requirements: *GCE:* 180-240. *IB:* 24. *BTEC NC:* DM. *BTEC ND:* MMM.

S75 THE UNIVERSITY OF STIRLING

STIRLING FK9 4LA

t: 01786 467044 f: 01786 466800
e: admissions@stir.ac.uk
// www.stir.ac.uk

NC16 BA Business Studies and Sports Studies

Duration: 4FT Hon

Entry Requirements: *GCE:* BCC. *SQAH:* BBBB. *SQAAH:* AAA-CCC. *BTEC ND:* DMM.

S82 UNIVERSITY CAMPUS SUFFOLK

WATERFRONT BUILDING
NEPTUNE QUAY
IPSWICH
SUFFOLK IP4 1QJ

t: 01473 338348 f: 01473 339900
e: info@ucs.ac.uk
// www.ucs.ac.uk

C603 FdA Sport & Physical Activity Development

Duration: 2FT Fdg

Entry Requirements: *GCE:* 160.

CL65 FdSc Sport, Health & Exercise

Duration: 2FT Fdg

Entry Requirements: *GCE:* 160. *IB:* 24. *BTEC NC:* PP. *BTEC ND:* PPP.

S84 UNIVERSITY OF SUNDERLAND

STUDENT HELPLINE
THE STUDENT GATEWAY
CHESTER ROAD
SUNDERLAND SR1 3SD

t: 0191 515 3000 f: 0191 515 3805
e: student-helpline@sunderland.ac.uk
// www.sunderland.ac.uk

M9C6 BA Criminology with Sport

Duration: 3FT Hon

Entry Requirements: *GCE:* 220-360. *BTEC NC:* DM. *BTEC ND:* MMM. *OCR ND:* Distinction. *OCR NED:* Merit.

W5C6 BA Dance with Sport

Duration: 3FT Hon

Entry Requirements: *GCE:* 220-360. *BTEC NC:* DM. *BTEC ND:* MMM. *OCR ND:* Distinction. *OCR NED:* Merit.

Q3C6 BA English Studies with Sport

Duration: 3FT Hon

Entry Requirements: *GCE:* 220-360. *BTEC NC:* DM. *BTEC ND:* MMM. *OCR ND:* Distinction. *OCR NED:* Merit.

NC36 BA Financial Management and Sport

Duration: 3FT Hon

Entry Requirements: *GCE:* 220-360. *BTEC NC:* DM. *BTEC ND:* MMM. *OCR ND:* Distinction. *OCR NED:* Merit.

L7C6 BA Geography with Sport

Duration: 3FT Hon

Entry Requirements: *GCE:* 220-360. *BTEC NC:* DM. *BTEC ND:* MMM. *OCR ND:* Distinction. *OCR NED:* Merit.

V1C6 BA History with Sport

Duration: 3FT Hon

Entry Requirements: *GCE:* 220-360. *BTEC NC:* DM. *BTEC ND:* MMM. *OCR ND:* Distinction. *OCR NED:* Merit.

NC66 BA Human Resource Management and Sport

Duration: 3FT Hon

Entry Requirements: *GCE:* 220-360. *BTEC NC:* DM. *BTEC ND:* MMM. *OCR ND:* Distinction. *OCR NED:* Merit.

N6C6 BA Human Resource Management with Sport

Duration: 3FT Hon

Entry Requirements: *GCE:* 220-360. *BTEC NC:* DM. *BTEC ND:* MMM. *OCR ND:* Distinction. *OCR NED:* Merit.

CQ6H BA Sport and Modern Foreign Language (English)

Duration: 3FT Hon

Entry Requirements: *GCE:* 220-360. *BTEC NC:* DM. *BTEC ND:* MMM. *OCR ND:* Distinction. *OCR NED:* Merit.

C605 BA Sport Studies

Duration: 3FT Hon

Entry Requirements: *GCE:* 240-360. *IB:* 36. *BTEC NC:* DD. *BTEC ND:* MMM. *OCR ND:* Distinction. *OCR NED:* Merit.

C6N3 BA Sport with Financial Management

Duration: 3FT Hon

Entry Requirements: *GCE:* 220-360. *BTEC NC:* DM. *BTEC ND:* MMM. *OCR ND:* Distinction. *OCR NED:* Merit.

C6V1 BA Sport with History

Duration: 3FT Hon

Entry Requirements: *GCE:* 220-360. *BTEC NC:* DM. *BTEC ND:* MMM. *OCR ND:* Distinction. *OCR NED:* Merit.

C6QH BA Sport with Modern Foreign Languages (English)

Duration: 3FT Hon

Entry Requirements: *GCE:* 220-360. *BTEC NC:* DM. *BTEC ND:* MMM. *OCR ND:* Distinction. *OCR NED:* Merit.

CG64 BA/BSc Sport and Computing

Duration: 3FT Hon

Entry Requirements: *GCE:* 220-360. *BTEC NC:* DM. *BTEC ND:* MMM. *OCR ND:* Distinction. *OCR NED:* Merit.

CW65 BA/BSc Sport and Dance

Duration: 3FT Hon

Entry Requirements: *GCE:* 220-360. *BTEC NC:* DM. *BTEC ND:* MMM. *OCR ND:* Distinction. *OCR NED:* Merit.

CX63 BA/BSc Sport and Education

Duration: 3FT Hon

Entry Requirements: *GCE:* 220-360. *BTEC NC:* DM. *BTEC ND:* MMM. *OCR ND:* Distinction. *OCR NED:* Merit.

CQ61 BA/BSc Sport and English Language/Linguistics

Duration: 3FT Hon

Entry Requirements: *GCE:* 220-360. *BTEC NC:* DM. *BTEC ND:* MMM. *OCR ND:* Distinction. *OCR NED:* Merit.

CL67 BA/BSc Sport and Geography

Duration: 3FT Hon

Entry Requirements: *GCE:* 220-360. *BTEC NC:* DM. *BTEC ND:* MMM. *OCR ND:* Distinction. *OCR NED:* Merit.

CW63 BA/BSc Sport and Music

Duration: 3FT Hon

Entry Requirements: *GCE:* 220-360. *BTEC NC:* DM. *BTEC ND:* MMM. *OCR ND:* Distinction. *OCR NED:* Merit.

CW66 BA/BSc Sport and Photography

Duration: 3FT Hon

Entry Requirements: *GCE:* 220-360. *BTEC NC:* DM. *BTEC ND:* MMM. *OCR ND:* Distinction. *OCR NED:* Merit.

CL62 BA/BSc Sport and Politics

Duration: 3FT Hon

Entry Requirements: *GCE:* 220-360. *BTEC NC:* DM. *BTEC ND:* MMM. *OCR ND:* Distinction. *OCR NED:* Merit.

C6R2 BA/BSc Sport with Modern Foreign Languages (German)

Duration: 3FT Hon

Entry Requirements: *GCE:* 220-360. *BTEC NC:* DM. *BTEC ND:* MMM. *OCR ND:* Distinction. *OCR NED:* Merit.

C8C6 BSc Psychology with Sport

Duration: 3FT Hon

Entry Requirements: *GCE:* 220-360. *BTEC NC:* DM. *BTEC ND:* MMM. *OCR ND:* Distinction. *OCR NED:* Merit.

C602 BSc Sport and Exercise Development

Duration: 4SW Hon

Entry Requirements: *GCE:* 240-360. *IB:* 36. *BTEC NC:* DD. *BTEC ND:* MMM. *OCR ND:* Distinction. *OCR NED:* Merit.

C603 BSc Sport and Exercise Development (Foundation)

Duration: 4FT Hon

Entry Requirements: *GCE:* 100-360. *SQAH:* CC.

C601 BSc Sport and Exercise Sciences

Duration: 3FT Hon

Entry Requirements: *GCE:* 240-360. *IB:* 36. *BTEC NC:* DD. *BTEC ND:* MMM. *OCR ND:* Distinction. *OCR NED:* Merit.

C6T7 BSc Sport with American Studies

Duration: 3FT Hon

Entry Requirements: *GCE:* 220-360. *BTEC NC:* DM. *BTEC ND:* MMM. *OCR ND:* Distinction. *OCR NED:* Merit.

C6B9 BSc Sport with Community Health

Duration: 3FT Hon

Entry Requirements: *GCE:* 220-360. *BTEC NC:* DM. *BTEC ND:* MMM. *OCR ND:* Distinction. *OCR NED:* Merit.

C6W5 BSc Sport with Dance
Duration: 3FT Hon

Entry Requirements: *GCE:* 220-360. *BTEC NC:* DM. *BTEC ND:* MMM. *OCR ND:* Distinction. *OCR NED:* Merit.

C6X3 BSc Sport with Education
Duration: 3FT Hon

Entry Requirements: *GCE:* 220-360. *BTEC NC:* DM. *BTEC ND:* MMM. *OCR ND:* Distinction. *OCR NED:* Merit.

C6W3 BSc Sport with Music
Duration: 3FT Hon

Entry Requirements: *GCE:* 220-360. *BTEC NC:* DM. *BTEC ND:* MMM. *OCR ND:* Distinction. *OCR NED:* Merit.

C6L3 BSc Sport with Sociology
Duration: 3FT Hon

Entry Requirements: *GCE:* 220-360. *BTEC NC:* DM. *BTEC ND:* MMM. *OCR ND:* Distinction. *OCR NED:* Merit.

C606 FdSc Exercise, Health & Fitness
Duration: 2FT Fdg

Entry Requirements: *GCE:* 100-240. *BTEC NC:* MP. *BTEC ND:* PPP. *OCR ND:* Pass. *OCR NED:* Pass.

S93 SWANSEA UNIVERSITY
SINGLETON PARK
SWANSEA SA2 8PP
t: 01792 295111 f: 01792 295110
e: admissions@swansea.ac.uk
// www.swansea.ac.uk

G1C6 BSc Mathematics with Sports Science
Duration: 3FT Hon

Entry Requirements: *GCE:* 280.

F3C6 BSc Physics with Sports Science
Duration: 3FT Hon

Entry Requirements: *GCE:* 260-280. *SQAH:* AABCC. *SQAAH:* BCC.

T20 UNIVERSITY OF TEESSIDE
MIDDLESBROUGH TS1 3BA
t: 01642 218121 f: 01642 384201
e: registry@tees.ac.uk
// www.tees.ac.uk

CX69 FdA Outdoor Leadership
Duration: 2FT Fdg

Entry Requirements: *GCE:* 120.

T80 TRINITY UNIVERSITY COLLEGE (PREVIOUSLY TRINITY COLLEGE CARMARTHEN)
COLLEGE ROAD
CARMARTHEN SA31 3EP
t: 01267 676767 f: 01267 676766
e: registry@trinity-cm.ac.uk
// www.trinity-cm.ac.uk/

BC46 BA Health & Exercise and Sports Studies
Duration: 3FT Hon

Entry Requirements: *GCE:* 180-360. *IB:* 26. *BTEC NC:* MM. *BTEC ND:* MMM. Interview required.

T85 TRURO AND PENWITH COLLEGE (FORMERLY TRURO COLLEGE)
TRURO COLLEGE
COLLEGE ROAD
TRURO
CORNWALL TR1 3XX
t: 01872 267122 f: 01872 267526
e: heinfo@trurocollege.ac.uk
// www.trurocollege.ac.uk

CN62 FdSc Sports Performance Analysis and Management
Duration: 2FT Fdg

Entry Requirements: Contact the institution for details.

T90 TYNE METROPOLITAN COLLEGE
EMBLETON AVENUE
WALLSEND
TYNE AND WEAR NE28 9NJ
t: 0191 229 5000 f: 0191 229 5301
e: enquiries@tynemet.ac.uk
// www.tynemet.ac.uk

C600 FdSc Sport (Exercise & Development)
Duration: 2FT Fdg

Entry Requirements: Interview required.

U20 UNIVERSITY OF ULSTER
COLERAINE
CO. LONDONDERRY
NORTHERN IRELAND BT52 1SA
t: 028 7032 4221 f: 028 7032 4908
e: online@ulster.ac.uk
// www.ulster.ac.uk

C602 BSc Sports Technology (with Integrated Foundation Year)
Duration: 5SW Hon

Entry Requirements: *GCE:* 120. *IB:* 24. *BTEC ND:* PPP.

U40 UNIVERSITY OF THE WEST OF SCOTLAND

PAISLEY
RENFREWSHIRE
SCOTLAND PA1 2BE

t: 0141 848 3727 f: 0141 848 3623
e: admissions@uws.ac.uk

// www.uws.ac.uk

CN62 BA Outdoor Recreation

Duration: 1FT/2FT Ord/Hon

Entry Requirements: HND required.

CB69 BSc Exercise & Health

Duration: 1FT/2FT Ord/Hon

Entry Requirements: HND required.

C601 DipHE Sport Development

Duration: 2FT Dip

Entry Requirements: *SQAH:* BBC.

W08 WAKEFIELD COLLEGE

MARGARET STREET
WAKEFIELD
WEST YORKSHIRE WF1 2DH

t: 01924 789111 f: 01924 789281
e: courseinfo@wakefield.ac.uk

// www.wakefield.ac.uk

C600 BSc Health Related Exercise and Fitness

Duration: 1FT Hon

Entry Requirements: *GCE:* 240.

W25 WARWICKSHIRE COLLEGE

WARWICK NEW ROAD
LEAMINGTON SPA
WARWICKSHIRE CV32 5JE

t: 01926 318 000 f: 01926 318 111
e: he@warkscol.ac.uk

// www.warkscol.ac.uk

62CN HND Sport & Leisure Management (Health and Fitness)

Duration: 2FT HND

Entry Requirements: *GCE:* 80.

W50 UNIVERSITY OF WESTMINSTER

115 NEW CAVENDISH STREET
LONDON W1W 6UW

t: 020 7911 5000 f: 020 7911 5788
e: course-enquiries@westminster.ac.uk

// www.westminster.ac.uk

BC46 BSc Nutrition and Exercise Science

Duration: 3FT Hon

Entry Requirements: *GCE:* CCD. *SQAH:* CCCC. *IB:* 26. *BTEC NC:* DM. *BTEC ND:* MMP.

BCK6 BSc Nutrition and Exercise Science with Foundation

Duration: 4FT Hon

Entry Requirements: *GCE:* CC. *SQAH:* CCCC. *IB:* 26. *BTEC NC:* MM. *BTEC ND:* MPP. Interview required.

W67 WIGAN AND LEIGH COLLEGE

PO BOX 53
PARSONS WALK
WIGAN WN1 1RS

t: 01942 761605 f: 01942 760223

// www.wigan-leigh.ac.uk

CN68 FdA Exercise & Fitness Management

Duration: 2FT Fdg

Entry Requirements: Interview required.

W75 UNIVERSITY OF WOLVERHAMPTON

ADMISSIONS UNIT
MX207, CAMP STREET
WOLVERHAMPTON
WEST MIDLANDS WV1 1AD

t: 01902 321000 f: 01902 321896
e: admissions@wlv.ac.uk

// www.wlv.ac.uk

NCV6 BA Event & Venue Management and Sports Studies

Duration: 3FT Hon

Entry Requirements: *GCE:* 160-220.

LC36 BA Sociology and Sports Studies

Duration: 3FT Hon

Entry Requirements: *GCE:* 160-220.

C601 BA Sports Studies

Duration: 3FT Hon

Entry Requirements: *GCE:* 160-220.

CW65 BA Sports Studies and Dance Practice & Performance

Duration: 3FT Hon

Entry Requirements: *GCE:* 160-220.

CV61 BA Sports Studies and History

Duration: 3FT Hon

Entry Requirements: *GCE:* 160-220. *IB:* 24.

C600 FdSc Sport and Exercise Science

Duration: 2FT Fdg

Entry Requirements: *GCE:* 80-140.

W76 UNIVERSITY OF WINCHESTER

WINCHESTER
HANTS SO22 4NR

t: 01962 827234 f: 01962 827288
e: course.enquiries@winchester.ac.uk

// www.winchester.ac.uk

LC5Q BA Childhood, Youth & Community Studies and Sports Studies

Duration: 3FT Hon

Entry Requirements: *Foundation:* Pass. *GCE:* 220-260. *IB:* 26. *BTEC NC:* DD. *BTEC ND:* MMP. *OCR ND:* Distinction.

WC6P BA Film & Cinema Technologies and Sports Studies

Duration: 3FT Deg

Entry Requirements: *Foundation:* Pass. *GCE:* 220-260. *IB:* 26. *BTEC NC:* DD. *BTEC ND:* MMP. *OCR ND:* Distinction.

MC16 BA Law and Sports Studies

Duration: 3FT Hon

Entry Requirements: *Foundation:* Merit. *GCE:* 220-280. *IB:* 24. *BTEC NC:* DM. *BTEC ND:* MMP.

C600 BA Sports Studies

Duration: 3FT Hon

Entry Requirements: *Foundation:* Merit. *GCE:* 220-280. *IB:* 24. *BTEC NC:* DM. *BTEC ND:* MMP.

TCR6 DipHE American Literature and Sports Studies

Duration: 2FT Dip

Entry Requirements: *Foundation:* Pass. *GCE:* 120. *IB:* 20. *BTEC NC:* MP. *BTEC ND:* PPP.

VC46 DipHE Ancient & Medieval Archaeology & Art and Sports Studies

Duration: 2FT Dip

Entry Requirements: *Foundation:* Pass. *GCE:* 120. *IB:* 20. *BTEC NC:* MP. *BTEC ND:* PPP.

LCM6 DipHE Childhood, Youth & Community Studies and Sports Studies

Duration: 2FT Dip

Entry Requirements: *Foundation:* Pass. *GCE:* 120. *IB:* 20. *BTEC NC:* MP. *BTEC ND:* PPP.

VCP6 DipHE Ethics & Spirituality and Sports Studies

Duration: 2FT Dip

Entry Requirements: *Foundation:* Pass. *GCE:* 120. *IB:* 20. *BTEC NC:* MP. *BTEC ND:* PPP.

NCW6 DipHE Event Management and Sports Studies

Duration: 2FT Dip

Entry Requirements: *Foundation:* Pass. *GCE:* 120. *IB:* 20. *BTEC NC:* MP. *BTEC ND:* PPP.

CW63 DipHE Sports Studies and Vocal & Choral Studies

Duration: 2FT Dip

Entry Requirements: *Foundation:* Pass. *GCE:* 120. *IB:* 20. *BTEC NC:* MP. *BTEC ND:* PPP.

W80 UNIVERSITY OF WORCESTER

HENWICK GROVE
WORCESTER WR2 6AJ

t: 01905 855111 f: 01905 855377
e: admissions@worc.ac.uk

// www.worcester.ac.uk

CT67 BA/BSc American Studies and Sports Studies

Duration: 3FT Hon

Entry Requirements: *GCE:* 240-260. *IB:* 24. *BTEC NC:* DD. *BTEC ND:* MMM. *OCR ND:* Distinction. *OCR NED:* Merit.

QC3P BA/BSc English Language Studies and Sports Studies

Duration: 3FT Hon

Entry Requirements: *GCE:* 240-260. *IB:* 24. *BTEC NC:* DD. *BTEC ND:* MMM. *OCR ND:* Distinction. *OCR NED:* Merit.

QC36 BA/BSc English Literary Studies and Sports Studies

Duration: 3FT Hon

Entry Requirements: *GCE:* 240-260. *IB:* 24. *BTEC NC:* DD. *BTEC ND:* MMM. *OCR ND:* Distinction. *OCR NED:* Merit.

LC2P BA/BSc Politics: People & Power and Sports Studies

Duration: 3FT Hon

Entry Requirements: *GCE:* 240-260. *IB:* 24. *BTEC NC:* DD. *BTEC ND:* MMM. *OCR ND:* Distinction. *OCR NED:* Merit.

LC36 BA/BSc Sociology and Sports Studies

Duration: 3FT Hon

Entry Requirements: *GCE:* 240-260. *IB:* 24. *BTEC NC:* DD. *BTEC ND:* MMM. *OCR ND:* Distinction. *OCR NED:* Merit.

CC26 BSc Animal Biology and Sports Studies

Duration: 3FT Hon

Entry Requirements: *GCE:* 240. *IB:* 24. *BTEC ND:* DMM. *OCR ND:* Distinction. *OCR NED:* Merit.

BC4P BSc Human Nutrition and Sports Studies

Duration: 3FT Hon

Entry Requirements: *GCE:* 240. *IB:* 24. *BTEC ND:* DMM. *OCR ND:* Distinction. *OCR NED:* Merit.

C691 BSc Physical Education and Sports Studies

Duration: 3FT Hon

Entry Requirements: *GCE:* 240. *IB:* 24. *BTEC NC:* DD. *BTEC ND:* MMM. *OCR ND:* Distinction. *OCR NED:* Merit.

CF6V BSc Physical Geography and Sports Studies

Duration: 3FT Hon

Entry Requirements: *GCE:* 240-260. *IB:* 24. *BTEC NC:* DD. *BTEC ND:* MMM. *OCR ND:* Distinction. *OCR NED:* Merit.

006C HND Sports Studies

Duration: 2FT HND

Entry Requirements: *GCE:* 300.

W85 WRITTLE COLLEGE

REGISTRY
WRITTLE COLLEGE
CHELMSFORD
ESSEX CM1 3RR

t: 01245 424200 **f:** 01245 420456
e: admissions@writtle.ac.uk

// www.writtle.ac.uk

C600 BSc Sports and Exercise Performance

Duration: 3FT/4SW Hon

Entry Requirements: HND required.

Y75 YORK ST JOHN UNIVERSITY

LORD MAYOR'S WALK
YORK YO31 7EX

t: 01904 876598 **f:** 01904 876940/876921
e: admissions@yorksj.ac.uk

// www.yorksj.ac.uk

NC2P BA Business Management and Sport, Society & Development

Duration: 3FT Hon

Entry Requirements: Contact the institution for details.

CL66 BA Sport, Society & Development

Duration: 3FT Hon

Entry Requirements: Contact the institution for details.

SPORTS THERAPY

B16 UNIVERSITY OF BATH

CLAVERTON DOWN
BATH BA2 7AY

t: 01225 383019 **f:** 01225 386366
e: admissions@bath.ac.uk

// www.bath.ac.uk

CB69 FdSc Sport (Sports Therapy)

Duration: 2FT Fdg

Entry Requirements: *GCE:* 80.

B22 UNIVERSITY OF BEDFORDSHIRE

PARK SQUARE
LUTON
BEDS LU1 3JU

t: 01582 489286 **f:** 01582 489323
e: admissions@beds.ac.uk

// www.beds.ac.uk

CB63 BSc Sports Therapy

Duration: 3FT Hon

Entry Requirements: *GCE:* 160-240. *SQAH:* BCC. *SQAAH:* BB. *IB:* 30.

C605 FdSc Sports Therapy

Duration: 2FT Fdg

Entry Requirements: Contact the institution for details.

B35 UNIVERSITY COLLEGE BIRMINGHAM
SUMMER ROW
BIRMINGHAM B3 1JB
t: 0121 604 1040 **f:** 0121 604 1166
e: admissions@ucb.ac.uk
// www.ucb.ac.uk

C600 BSc Sports Therapy
Duration: 3FT Hon

Entry Requirements: *GCE:* 100.

C602 FdSc Sports Therapy
Duration: 2FT Fdg

Entry Requirements: *GCE:* 100.

B44 THE UNIVERSITY OF BOLTON
DEANE ROAD
BOLTON BL3 5AB
t: 01204 900600 **f:** 01204 399074
e: enquiries@bolton.ac.uk
// www.bolton.ac.uk

C602 BSc Sports Rehabilitation
Duration: 3FT Hon

Entry Requirements: *GCE:* 240. *IB:* 24. *BTEC ND:* MMM.

C20 UNIVERSITY OF WALES INSTITUTE, CARDIFF
PO BOX 377
LLANDAFF CAMPUS
WESTERN AVENUE
CARDIFF CF5 2SG
t: 029 2041 6070 **f:** 029 2041 6286
e: admissions@uwic.ac.uk
// www.uwic.ac.uk

C607 BSc Sport Conditioning, Rehabilitation and Massage
Duration: 3FT Hon

Entry Requirements: *GCE:* 300. *IB:* 25. *BTEC ND:* DDM.

C85 COVENTRY UNIVERSITY
THE STUDENT CENTRE
COVENTRY UNIVERSITY
1 GULSON RD
COVENTRY CV1 2JH
t: 024 7615 2222 **f:** 024 7615 2223
e: studentenquiries@coventry.ac.uk
// www.coventry.ac.uk

BC96 BSc Sports Therapy
Duration: 3FT/4SW Hon

Entry Requirements: *GCE:* 260. *BTEC ND:* DMM.

C99 UNIVERSITY OF CUMBRIA
FUSEHILL STREET
CARLISLE
CUMBRIA CA1 2HH
t: 01228 616234 **f:** 01228 616235
// www.cumbria.ac.uk

CB69 BSc Sport & Exercise Therapy
Duration: 3FT Hon

Entry Requirements: Contact the institution for details.

CB63 FdSc Sport Therapy and Massage
Duration: 2FT Fdg

Entry Requirements: HND required.

D39 UNIVERSITY OF DERBY
KEDLESTON ROAD
DERBY DE22 1GB
t: 08701 202330 **f:** 01332 597724
e: askadmissions@derby.ac.uk
// www.derby.ac.uk

C690 BA Physical Activity & Health and Sports Massage & Exercise Therapy
Duration: 3FT Hon

Entry Requirements: *Foundation:* Merit. *GCE:* 160-240. *IB:* 26. *BTEC NC:* MM. *BTEC ND:* MMP.

C611 BA Sports Massage & Exercise Therapy and Sports Development
Duration: 3FT Hon

Entry Requirements: *Foundation:* Merit. *GCE:* 160-240. *IB:* 26. *BTEC NC:* MM. *BTEC ND:* MMP.

BCH6 BA/BSc Spa Therapies and Sports Massage & Exercise Therapies
Duration: 3FT Hon

Entry Requirements: *Foundation:* Merit. *GCE:* 160-240. *IB:* 26. *BTEC NC:* MM. *BTEC ND:* MMP.

C608 BA/BSc Sports Massage & Exercise Therapy and Martial Arts Theory & Practice
Duration: 3FT Hon

Entry Requirements: *Foundation:* Merit. *GCE:* 160-240. *IB:* 26. *BTEC NC:* MM. *BTEC ND:* MMP.

E81 EXETER COLLEGE

HELE ROAD
EXETER
DEVON EX4 4JS

t: 01392 205582 **f:** 01392 279972
e: ebs@exe-coll.ac.uk
// www.exe-coll.ac.uk

BC36 FdSc Sports Therapy

Duration: 2FT Fdg

Entry Requirements: Contact the institution for details.

G50 THE UNIVERSITY OF GLOUCESTERSHIRE

HARDWICK CAMPUS
ST PAUL'S ROAD
CHELTENHAM GL50 4BS

t: 01242 714501 **f:** 01242 543334
e: admissions@glos.ac.uk
// www.glos.ac.uk

C606 BSc Sports Therapy

Duration: 3FT Hon

Entry Requirements: HND required.

H36 UNIVERSITY OF HERTFORDSHIRE

UNIVERSITY ADMISSIONS SERVICE
COLLEGE LANE
HATFIELD
HERTS AL10 9AB

t: 01707 284800 **f:** 01707 284870
// www.herts.ac.uk

CB63 BSc Sports Therapy

Duration: 3FT Hon

Entry Requirements: *GCE:* 260.

H72 THE UNIVERSITY OF HULL

THE UNIVERSITY OF HULL
COTTINGHAM ROAD
HULL HU6 7RX

t: 01482 466100 **f:** 01482 442290
e: admissions@hull.ac.uk
// www.hull.ac.uk

C602 BSc Sports Rehabilitation

Duration: 3FT Hon

Entry Requirements: *GCE:* 240-280. *IB:* 30.

L68 LONDON METROPOLITAN UNIVERSITY

166-220 HOLLOWAY ROAD
LONDON N7 8DB

t: 020 7133 4200
e: admissions@londonmet.ac.uk
// www.londonmet.ac.uk

CW65 BSc Sport & Dance Therapy

Duration: 3FT Hon

Entry Requirements: *GCE:* 240. *IB:* 28. *BTEC ND:* MMM.

CB63 BSc Sports Therapy

Duration: 3FT Hon

Entry Requirements: *GCE:* 280. *IB:* 28.

C605 FdSc Personal Training & Fitness Consultancy

Duration: 2FT Fdg

Entry Requirements: Contact the institution for details.

N23 NEWCASTLE COLLEGE

STUDENT SERVICES
RYE HILL CAMPUS
SCOTSWOOD ROAD
NEWCASTLE UPON TYNE NE4 7SA

t: 0191 200 4000 **f:** 0191 200 4349
e: enquiries@ncl-coll.ac.uk
// www.newcastlecollege.co.uk

CB6X BSc Sports Therapy (Top-up)

Duration: 1FT Hon

Entry Requirements: HND required.

N38 UNIVERSITY OF NORTHAMPTON

PARK CAMPUS
BOUGHTON GREEN ROAD
NORTHAMPTON NN2 7AL

t: 0800 358 2232 **f:** 01604 722083
e: admissions@northampton.ac.uk
// www.northampton.ac.uk

C605 BSc Sports Therapy (top-up)

Duration: 1FT Hon

Entry Requirements: HND required.

C601 FdSc Sports Therapy

Duration: 2FT Fdg

Entry Requirements: *GCE:* 40-80. *SQAH:* CC-BC. *IB:* 24.

N49 NESCOT, SURREY

REIGATE ROAD
EWELL
EPSOM
SURREY KT17 3DS

t: 020 8394 3038 **f:** 020 8394 3030
e: info@nescot.ac.uk

// www.nescot.ac.uk

C600 FdSc Sports Therapy

Duration: 2FT Fdg

Entry Requirements: *GCE:* CC. *BTEC ND:* MPP.

P60 UNIVERSITY OF PLYMOUTH

DRAKE CIRCUS
PLYMOUTH PL4 8AA

t: 01752 588037 **f:** 01752 588050
e: admissions@plymouth.ac.uk

// www.plymouth.ac.uk

C604 FdSc Sports Therapy

Duration: 2FT Fdg

Entry Requirements: *GCE:* 200.

P63 UCP MARJON - UNIVERSITY COLLEGE PLYMOUTH ST MARK & ST JOHN

DERRIFORD ROAD
PLYMOUTH PL6 8BH

t: 01752 636890 **f:** 01752 636819
e: admissions@marjon.ac.uk

// www.ucpmarjon.ac.uk

C607 BSc Sports Therapy

Duration: 1FT Hon

Entry Requirements: *GCE:* 180.

S03 THE UNIVERSITY OF SALFORD

SALFORD M5 4WT

t: 0161 295 4545 **f:** 0161 295 3126
e: ugadmissions-exrel@salford.ac.uk

// www.salford.ac.uk

BC96 BSc Sports Rehabilitation

Duration: 3FT Hon

Entry Requirements: *GCE:* 300. *SQAH:* AABBB. *SQAAH:* BBB. *IB:* 29. *BTEC ND:* DDM.

S28 SOMERSET COLLEGE OF ARTS AND TECHNOLOGY

WELLINGTON ROAD
TAUNTON
SOMERSET TA1 5AX

t: 01823 366331 **f:** 01823 366418
e: enquiries@somerset.ac.uk

// www.somerset.ac.uk/student-area/considering-a-degree.html

C601 FdSc Sports & Exercise Rehabilitation

Duration: 2FT Fdg

Entry Requirements: *GCE:* 80. *IB:* 24. *BTEC NC:* PP. *BTEC ND:* PPP.

S64 ST MARY'S UNIVERSITY COLLEGE, TWICKENHAM

WALDEGRAVE ROAD
STRAWBERRY HILL
MIDDLESEX TW1 4SX

t: 020 8240 4029 **f:** 020 8240 2361
e: admit@smuc.ac.uk

// www.smuc.ac.uk

C602 BSc Sport Rehabilitation

Duration: 3FT Hon

Entry Requirements: *GCE:* 180-200. *BTEC NC:* MM. *BTEC ND:* MPP. Interview required.

S72 STAFFORDSHIRE UNIVERSITY

COLLEGE ROAD
STOKE ON TRENT ST4 2DE

t: 01782 292753 **f:** 01782 292740
e: admissions@staffs.ac.uk

// www.staffs.ac.uk

BC96 BSc Sports Therapy

Duration: 3FT Hon

Entry Requirements: *GCE:* 180-240. *IB:* 24. *BTEC NC:* DM. *BTEC ND:* MMM.

T20 UNIVERSITY OF TEESSIDE

MIDDLESBROUGH TS1 3BA

t: 01642 218121 **f:** 01642 384201
e: registry@tees.ac.uk

// www.tees.ac.uk

C601 BSc Sports Therapy

Duration: 3FT Hon

Entry Requirements: *GCE:* 280.

U40 UNIVERSITY OF THE WEST OF SCOTLAND

PAISLEY
RENFREWSHIRE
SCOTLAND PA1 2BE

t: 0141 848 3727 f: 0141 848 3623
e: admissions@uws.ac.uk
// www.uws.ac.uk

BC96 BSc Sports Therapy

Duration: 1FT/2FT Ord/Hon

Entry Requirements: HND required.

W80 UNIVERSITY OF WORCESTER

HENWICK GROVE
WORCESTER WR2 6AJ

t: 01905 855111 f: 01905 855377
e: admissions@worc.ac.uk
// www.worcester.ac.uk

C603 BSc Sports Therapy

Duration: 3FT Hon

Entry Requirements: *GCE:* 260. *IB:* 24. *BTEC NC:* DD. *BTEC ND:* MMM. *OCR ND:* Distinction. *OCR NED:* Merit.

Y70 YORK COLLEGE

SIM BALK LANE
YORK YO23 2BB

t: 01904 770433 f: 01904 770499
e: adagorne@yorkcollege.ac.uk
// www.yorkcollege.ac.uk

C600 FdSc Sports Therapy

Duration: 2FT Fdg

Entry Requirements: *GCE:* CC. *BTEC NC:* MM. *BTEC ND:* MPP. Interview required.

SPORTS EDUCATION

B06 BANGOR UNIVERSITY

BANGOR
GWYNEDD LL57 2DG

t: 01248 382016/2017 f: 01248 370451
e: admissions@bangor.ac.uk
// www.bangor.ac.uk

CR63 BA Italian/Physical Education (4 years)

Duration: 4FT Hon

Entry Requirements: *GCE:* 260-280. *IB:* 28.

RC16 BA Physical Education/French (4 years)

Duration: 4FT Hon

Entry Requirements: *GCE:* 260-280. *IB:* 28.

QC16 BA Physical Education/Linguistics

Duration: 3FT Hon

Entry Requirements: *GCE:* 260-280. *IB:* 28.

FC16 BSc Chemistry/Physical Education

Duration: 3FT Hon

Entry Requirements: *GCE:* 260-280. *IB:* 28.

RC1P BSc Physical Education/French

Duration: 4FT Hon

Entry Requirements: *GCE:* 260-280. *IB:* 28.

RC4P BSc Physical Education/Spanish

Duration: 4FT Hon

Entry Requirements: *GCE:* 260-280. *IB:* 28.

C651 BSc Sport, Health & Physical Education

Duration: 3FT Hon

Entry Requirements: *GCE:* 260-280. *IB:* 28.

B16 UNIVERSITY OF BATH

CLAVERTON DOWN
BATH BA2 7AY

t: 01225 383019 f: 01225 386366
e: admissions@bath.ac.uk
// www.bath.ac.uk

CX63 BA Coach Education and Sports Development

Duration: 3FT Hon

Entry Requirements: *GCE:* AAB. *SQAAH:* ABB.

CX6H BA Coach Education and Sports Development with Placement

Duration: 4SW Hon

Entry Requirements: *GCE:* AAB. *SQAAH:* ABB.

CX6C BSc Sport (Coaching) (Work-based Learning)

Duration: 1FT Ord

Entry Requirements: Contact the institution for details.

B22 UNIVERSITY OF BEDFORDSHIRE

PARK SQUARE
LUTON
BEDS LU1 3JU

t: 01582 489286 f: 01582 489323
e: admissions@beds.ac.uk

// www.beds.ac.uk

X1C6 BA Physical Education - Secondary

Duration: 4FT Hon

Entry Requirements: *GCE:* 220-320. Interview required.

C601 BA Sport and Physical Education

Duration: 3FT Hon

Entry Requirements: Contact the institution for details.

C609 FdA Health, Fitness & Personal Training

Duration: 2FT Fdg

Entry Requirements: Contact the institution for details.

B38 BISHOP GROSSETESTE UNIVERSITY COLLEGE LINCOLN

LINCOLN LN1 3DY

t: 01522 583658 f: 01522 530243
e: info@bishopg.ac.uk

// www.bishopg.ac.uk

CX63 BA Education Studies/Sport

Duration: 3FT Hon

Entry Requirements: *GCE:* 160. Interview required.

X1FA BSc Education Studies/Science

Duration: 3FT Hon

Entry Requirements: *GCE:* 160.

B72 UNIVERSITY OF BRIGHTON

MITHRAS HOUSE
LEWES ROAD
BRIGHTON BN2 4AT

t: 01273 644644 f: 01273 642607
e: admissions@brighton.ac.uk

// www.brighton.ac.uk

X1C6 BA Physical Education with QTS (Secondary) (4 years)

Duration: 4FT Hon

Entry Requirements: Interview required.

C20 UNIVERSITY OF WALES INSTITUTE, CARDIFF

PO BOX 377
LLANDAFF CAMPUS
WESTERN AVENUE
CARDIFF CF5 2SG

t: 029 2041 6070 f: 029 2041 6286
e: admissions@uwic.ac.uk

// www.uwic.ac.uk

XB39 BA Educational Studies and Sport & Physical Activity

Duration: 3FT Hon

Entry Requirements: *GCE:* 260. *IB:* 24. *BTEC ND:* DMM. *OCR NED:* Merit.

C58 UNIVERSITY OF CHICHESTER

BISHOP OTTER CAMPUS
COLLEGE LANE
CHICHESTER
WEST SUSSEX PO19 6PE

t: 01243 816002 f: 01243 816161
e: admissions@chi.ac.uk

// www.chiuni.ac.uk

XC16 BA Physical Education and Teaching (Secondary) (4-year course)

Duration: 4FT Hon

Entry Requirements: *GCE:* 240-360. *IB:* 24. *BTEC NC:* DD. *BTEC ND:* MMM. Interview required.

C99 UNIVERSITY OF CUMBRIA

FUSEHILL STREET
CARLISLE
CUMBRIA CA1 2HH

t: 01228 616234 f: 01228 616235

// www.cumbria.ac.uk

XCC6 BA Physical Education

Duration: 3FT Hon

Entry Requirements: *Foundation:* Pass. *GCE:* 200. *IB:* 32. *BTEC NC:* DM. *BTEC ND:* MMP.

D39 UNIVERSITY OF DERBY

KEDLESTON ROAD
DERBY DE22 1GB

t: 08701 202330 f: 01332 597724
e: askadmissions@derby.ac.uk

// www.derby.ac.uk

CL64 BA Martial Arts Theory & Practice and Public Services Management

Duration: 3FT Hon

Entry Requirements: *Foundation:* Merit. *GCE:* 160-240. *IB:* 26. *BTEC NC:* MM. *BTEC ND:* MMP.

E14 UNIVERSITY OF EAST ANGLIA

NORWICH NR4 7TJ

t: 01603 456161 f: 01603 458596
e: admissions@uea.ac.uk

// www.uea.ac.uk

XC16 BA Physical Education and Sport

Duration: 3FT Hon

Entry Requirements: Contact the institution for details.

E42 EDGE HILL UNIVERSITY

ORMSKIRK
LANCASHIRE L39 4QP

t: 0800 195 5063 f: 01695 584355
e: enquiries@edgehill.ac.uk

// www.edgehill.ac.uk

C605 BA Coach Education

Duration: 3FT Hon

Entry Requirements: *GCE:* 240. *IB:* 28. *BTEC NC:* DD. *BTEC ND:* MMM. *OCR ND:* Distinction.

L24 LEEDS TRINITY & ALL SAINTS (ACCREDITED COLLEGE OF THE UNIVERSITY OF LEEDS)

BROWNBERRIE LANE
HORSFORTH
LEEDS LS18 5HD

t: 0113 283 7150 f: 0113 283 7222
e: enquiries@leedstrinity.ac.uk

// www.leedstrinity.ac.uk

CX61 BA Physical Education (Primary) and Sports Development

Duration: 3FT Hon

Entry Requirements: *GCE:* 240. *IB:* 24. *BTEC NC:* PP. *BTEC ND:* PPP.

L51 LIVERPOOL JOHN MOORES UNIVERSITY

ROSCOE COURT
4 RODNEY STREET
LIVERPOOL L1 2TZ

t: 0151 231 5090 f: 0151 231 3462
e: recruitment@ljmu.ac.uk

// www.ljmu.ac.uk

X9CP BA Outdoor Education with Physical Education

Duration: 3FT Hon

Entry Requirements: *GCE:* 240.

XC1P BA Primary & Secondary Education: Physical Education

Duration: 3FT Hon

Entry Requirements: *GCE:* 220.

CXP3 BA Sport Development and Physical Education

Duration: 3FT Hon

Entry Requirements: *GCE:* 240. *BTEC ND:* MMM.

P63 UCP MARJON - UNIVERSITY COLLEGE PLYMOUTH ST MARK & ST JOHN

DERRIFORD ROAD
PLYMOUTH PL6 8BH

t: 01752 636890 f: 01752 636819
e: admissions@marjon.ac.uk

// www.ucpmarjon.ac.uk

CX6H BA Children's Physical Education

Duration: 3FT Hon

Entry Requirements: *GCE:* 220.

R48 ROEHAMPTON UNIVERSITY

ERASMUS HOUSE
ROEHAMPTON LANE
LONDON SW15 5PU

t: 020 8392 3232 f: 020 8392 3470
e: enquiries@roehampton.ac.uk

// www.roehampton.ac.uk

XCC6 BA Primary Education Foundation Stage & Key Stage 1 (Physical Education)

Duration: 3FT Hon

Entry Requirements: *GCE:* 300-360. *IB:* 25. *BTEC NC:* DD. *BTEC ND:* DDM. *OCR ND:* Distinction. *OCR NED:* Distinction. Interview required.

S21 SHEFFIELD HALLAM UNIVERSITY

CITY CAMPUS
HOWARD STREET
SHEFFIELD S1 1WB

t: 0114 225 5555 f: 0114 225 2167
e: admissions@shu.ac.uk

// www.shu.ac.uk

C603 BSc Physical Education and Youth Sport

Duration: 3FT Hon

Entry Requirements: *GCE:* 260.

S64 ST MARY'S UNIVERSITY COLLEGE, TWICKENHAM

WALDEGRAVE ROAD
STRAWBERRY HILL
MIDDLESEX TW1 4SX

t: 020 8240 4029 f: 020 8240 2361
e: admit@smuc.ac.uk

// www.smuc.ac.uk

C900 BA PE in the Community

Duration: 3FT Hon
Entry Requirements: *GCE:* 160-200. *BTEC NC:* MM. *BTEC ND:* MPP.

CC69 BA/BSc PE in the Community and Sport Science

Duration: 3FT Hon

Entry Requirements: *GCE:* 160-200. *BTEC NC:* MM. *BTEC ND:* MPP.

W75 UNIVERSITY OF WOLVERHAMPTON

ADMISSIONS UNIT
MX207, CAMP STREET
WOLVERHAMPTON
WEST MIDLANDS WV1 1AD

t: 01902 321000 f: 01902 321896
e: admissions@wlv.ac.uk

// www.wlv.ac.uk

C603 BA Physical Education

Duration: 3FT Hon

Entry Requirements: *GCE:* 160-220.

W76 UNIVERSITY OF WINCHESTER

WINCHESTER
HANTS SO22 4NR

t: 01962 827234 f: 01962 827288
e: course.enquiries@winchester.ac.uk

// www.winchester.ac.uk

XCC6 BA Physical Education: Primary (4 years QTS)

Duration: 4FT Hon

Entry Requirements: *Foundation:* Distinction. *GCE:* 260-300. *IB:* 24. *BTEC NC:* DD. *BTEC ND:* MMM. Interview required.

W80 UNIVERSITY OF WORCESTER

HENWICK GROVE
WORCESTER WR2 6AJ

t: 01905 855111 f: 01905 855377
e: admissions@worc.ac.uk

// www.worcester.ac.uk

CCD6 BSc Human Biology and Physical Education

Duration: 3FT Hon

Entry Requirements: *GCE:* 240. *IB:* 24. *BTEC ND:* DMM. *OCR ND:* Distinction. *OCR NED:* Merit.

SPORTS COACHING

B16 UNIVERSITY OF BATH

CLAVERTON DOWN
BATH BA2 7AY

t: 01225 383019 f: 01225 386366
e: admissions@bath.ac.uk

// www.bath.ac.uk

C602 BSc Sports Performance (Work-based Learning)

Duration: 1FT Ord

Entry Requirements: Contact the institution for details.

B22 UNIVERSITY OF BEDFORDSHIRE

PARK SQUARE
LUTON
BEDS LU1 3JU

t: 01582 489286 f: 01582 489323
e: admissions@beds.ac.uk

// www.beds.ac.uk

C614 FdSc Sport and Personal Training

Duration: 2FT Fdg

Entry Requirements: Contact the institution for details.

B37 BISHOP BURTON COLLEGE

BISHOP BURTON
BEVERLEY
EAST YORKSHIRE HU17 8QG

t: 01964 553000 f: 01964 553101
e: enquiries@bishopburton.ac.uk

// www.bishopburton.ac.uk

CX61 BSc Sport Coaching Development and Fitness

Duration: 3FT Hon

Entry Requirements: Contact the institution for details.

XC16 FdSc Sport Coaching Development and Fitness

Duration: 2FT Fdg

Entry Requirements: Contact the institution for details.

B41 BLACKPOOL AND THE FYLDE COLLEGE AN ASSOCIATE COLLEGE OF LANCASTER UNIVERSITY

ASHFIELD ROAD
BISPHAM
BLACKPOOL
LANCS FY2 0HB

t: 01253 504346 **f:** 01253 356127
e: admissions@blackpool.ac.uk

// www.blackpool.ac.uk

CX6C FdSc Sports Coaching

Duration: 2FT Fdg

Entry Requirements: *GCE:* 40. *SQAH:* C. *SQAAH:* C. *BTEC NC:* PP. *BTEC ND:* PPP.

B44 THE UNIVERSITY OF BOLTON

DEANE ROAD
BOLTON BL3 5AB

t: 01204 900600 **f:** 01204 399074
e: enquiries@bolton.ac.uk

// www.bolton.ac.uk

C601 BA Sport Development

Duration: 3FT Hon

Entry Requirements: *GCE:* 200. *IB:* 20. *BTEC NC:* DM. *BTEC ND:* MMP.

B50 BOURNEMOUTH UNIVERSITY

TALBOT CAMPUS
FERN BARROW
POOLE
DORSET BH12 5BB

t: 01202 524111

// www.bournemouth.ac.uk

C600 BSc Sport Development & Coaching Sciences

Duration: 4SW Hon

Entry Requirements: *GCE:* 300.

CX6C BSc Sports Coaching and Development (Top-up)

Duration: 1FT Hon

Entry Requirements: *GCE:* 80.

B60 BRADFORD COLLEGE: AN ASSOCIATE COLLEGE OF LEEDS METROPOLITAN UNIVERSITY

GREAT HORTON ROAD
BRADFORD
WEST YORKSHIRE BD7 1AY

t: 01274 433333 **f:** 01274 433241
e: admissions@bradfordcollege.ac.uk

// www.bradfordcollege.ac.uk

CX6C FdSc Sports Coaching

Duration: 2FT Fdg

Entry Requirements: Contact the institution for details.

B72 UNIVERSITY OF BRIGHTON

MITHRAS HOUSE
LEWES ROAD
BRIGHTON BN2 4AT

t: 01273 644644 **f:** 01273 642607
e: admissions@brighton.ac.uk

// www.brighton.ac.uk

CXP1 BA Sport Coaching and Development (top-up)

Duration: 1FT Hon

Entry Requirements: HND required.

CX6C BSc Sport Coaching

Duration: 3FT Hon

Entry Requirements: *GCE:* BBC. *IB:* 30. *BTEC ND:* DMM.

B80 UNIVERSITY OF THE WEST OF ENGLAND, BRISTOL

FRENCHAY CAMPUS
COLDHARBOUR LANE
BRISTOL BS16 1QY

t: +44 (0)117 32 83333 **f:** +44 (0)117 32 82810
e: admissions@uwe.ac.uk

// www.uwe.ac.uk

C600 BSc Sports Coaching

Duration: 3FT Hon

Entry Requirements: *GCE:* 240-280.

C602 FdSc Sports Coaching

Duration: 2FT Fdg

Entry Requirements: *GCE:* 80-120.

B94 BUCKINGHAMSHIRE NEW UNIVERSITY

QUEEN ALEXANDRA ROAD
HIGH WYCOMBE
BUCKS HP11 2JZ

t: 0800 0565 660 f: 01494 605023
e: admissions@bucks.ac.uk

// www.bucks.ac.uk

NC2Q FdA Sports Management and Golf Studies

Duration: 2FT Fdg

Entry Requirements: *GCE:* 100-140.

C30 UNIVERSITY OF CENTRAL LANCASHIRE

PRESTON
LANCS PR1 2HE

t: 01772 201201 f: 01772 894954
e: uadmissions@uclan.ac.uk

// www.uclan.ac.uk

C615 BA Adventure Sports Coaching

Duration: 3FT Hon

Entry Requirements: *GCE:* 200-240. *IB:* 28. *OCR ND:* Distinction.

CX69 BA Sports Coaching

Duration: 3FT/4SW Hon

Entry Requirements: *GCE:* 240. *IB:* 28. *OCR ND:* Distinction.

CX61 BA Sports Coaching (by blended learning) - April start

Duration: 3FT Hon

Entry Requirements: *GCE:* 200-240. *IB:* 28. *OCR ND:* Distinction.

CXQ1 BA Sports Coaching (by blended learning) - Oct start

Duration: 3FT Hon

Entry Requirements: *GCE:* 200-240. *IB:* 28. *OCR ND:* Distinction.

C607 BSc Personal Fitness Training

Duration: 3FT Hon

Entry Requirements: *GCE:* 120.

C58 UNIVERSITY OF CHICHESTER

BISHOP OTTER CAMPUS
COLLEGE LANE
CHICHESTER
WEST SUSSEX PO19 6PE

t: 01243 816002 f: 01243 816161
e: admissions@chi.ac.uk

// www.chiuni.ac.uk

CX63 BA Sports Coaching and Physical Education

Duration: 3FT Hon

Entry Requirements: Contact the institution for details.

C69 CITY OF SUNDERLAND COLLEGE

BEDE CENTRE
DURHAM ROAD
SUNDERLAND SR3 4AH

t: 0191 511 6260 f: 0191 511 6380
e: highered.admissions@citysun.ac.uk

// www.citysun.ac.uk

C600 FdSc Sports Coaching

Duration: 2FT Fdg

Entry Requirements: *GCE:* 80.

C78 CORNWALL COLLEGE

POOL
REDRUTH
CORNWALL TR15 3RD

t: 01209 616161 f: 01209 611612
e: he.admissions@cornwall.ac.uk

// www.cornwall.ac.uk

C600 BSc Sports Performance and Coaching (top up)

Duration: 1FT Hon

Entry Requirements: Interview required. HND required.

C99 UNIVERSITY OF CUMBRIA

FUSEHILL STREET
CARLISLE
CUMBRIA CA1 2HH

t: 01228 616234 f: 01228 616235

// www.cumbria.ac.uk

XB19 FdA Football Coaching and Fitness

Duration: 2FT Fdg

Entry Requirements: *GCE:* 80. *BTEC NC:* PP. *BTEC ND:* PPP.

D22 DEARNE VALLEY COLLEGE

MANVERS PARK
WATH-UPON-DEARNE
ROTHERHAM S63 7EW

t: 01709 513101 f: 01709 513110
e: gjones@dearne-coll.ac.uk

// www.dearne-coll.ac.uk

C600 FdSc Sports Coaching (Performance & Participation)

Duration: 2FT Fdg

Entry Requirements: Contact the institution for details.

D39 UNIVERSITY OF DERBY

KEDLESTON ROAD
DERBY DE22 1GB

t: 08701 202330 **f:** 01332 597724
e: askadmissions@derby.ac.uk

// www.derby.ac.uk

CX6C BA/BSc Sports Coaching and Sports Development

Duration: 3FT Hon

Entry Requirements: *Foundation:* Merit. *GCE:* 160-240. *IB:* 26. *BTEC NC:* MM. *BTEC ND:* MMP.

XC16 BA/BSc Sports Coaching and Sports Massage & Exercise Therapies

Duration: 3FT Hon

Entry Requirements: *Foundation:* Merit. *GCE:* 160-240. *IB:* 26. *BTEC NC:* MM. *BTEC ND:* MMP.

D55 DUCHY COLLEGE

STOKE CLIMSLAND
CALLINGTON
CORNWALL PL17 8PB

t: 01579 372327 **f:** 01579 372200
e: uni@duchy.ac.uk

// www.duchy.ac.uk

CN68 FdSc Adventure Sports Coaching

Duration: 2FT Fdg

Entry Requirements: *GCE:* 100-120.

CX61 FdSc Sports Development & Coaching

Duration: 2FT Fdg

Entry Requirements: *GCE:* 100-120.

E14 UNIVERSITY OF EAST ANGLIA

NORWICH NR4 7TJ

t: 01603 456161 **f:** 01603 458596
e: admissions@uea.ac.uk

// www.uea.ac.uk

C600 FdSc Sports Coaching

Duration: 2FT Fdg

Entry Requirements: *GCE:* 140.

E25 EAST LANCASHIRE INSTITUTE OF HIGHER EDUCATION AT BLACKBURN COLLEGE

DUKE STREET
BLACKBURN BB2 1LH

t: 01254 292594 **f:** 01254 260749
e: he-admissions@blackburn.ac.uk

// www.elihe.ac.uk

BC96 FdA Health and Personal Training

Duration: 2FT Fdg

Entry Requirements: Contact the institution for details.

E28 UNIVERSITY OF EAST LONDON

DOCKLANDS CAMPUS
UNIVERSITY WAY
LONDON E16 2RD

t: 020 8223 2835 **f:** 020 8223 2978
e: admiss@uel.ac.uk

// www.uel.ac.uk

CG64 BA/BSc Sports Coaching/Multimedia

Duration: 3FT Hon

Entry Requirements: *GCE:* 200. *IB:* 24. *BTEC NC:* DM. *BTEC ND:* MMP.

C602 BSc Sports Coaching

Duration: 3FT Hon

Entry Requirements: *GCE:* 200. *IB:* 24. *BTEC NC:* DM. *BTEC ND:* MMP.

C603 BSc Sports Coaching (Extended)

Duration: 4FT Hon

Entry Requirements: *GCE:* 80.

C6C8 BSc Sports Coaching with Psychology

Duration: 3FT Hon

Entry Requirements: *GCE:* 200. *IB:* 24.

E42 EDGE HILL UNIVERSITY

ORMSKIRK
LANCASHIRE L39 4QP

t: 0800 195 5063 **f:** 01695 584355
e: enquiries@edgehill.ac.uk

// www.edgehill.ac.uk

CX61 FdSc Sports Coaching

Duration: 2FT Fdg

Entry Requirements: Contact the institution for details.

E81 EXETER COLLEGE

HELE ROAD
EXETER
DEVON EX4 4JS
t: 01392 205582 **f:** 01392 279972
e: ebs@exe-coll.ac.uk
// www.exe-coll.ac.uk

C600 FdSc Coaching and Fitness

Duration: 2FT Fdg

Entry Requirements: *GCE:* 80.

G14 UNIVERSITY OF GLAMORGAN, CARDIFF AND PONTYPRIDD

ENQUIRIES AND ADMISSIONS UNIT
PONTYPRIDD CF37 1DL
t: 0800 716925 **f:** 01443 654050
e: enquiries@glam.ac.uk
// www.glam.ac.uk

CX6D BSc Sports Coaching and Performance (Top-up)

Duration: 1FT Hon

Entry Requirements: Contact the institution for details.

CX69 FdSc Football Coaching and Performance

Duration: 2.5FT Fdg

Entry Requirements: *GCE:* 80-140. *IB:* 24. *BTEC NC:* PP. *BTEC ND:* PPP.

G45 GLOUCESTERSHIRE COLLEGE

PRINCESS ELIZABETH WAY
CHELTENHAM GL51 7SJ
t: 0845 155 2020 **f:** 01242 532023
e: info@gloscol.ac.uk
// www.gloscol.ac.uk

CX61 FdSc Sports Development and Coaching

Duration: 2FT Fdg

Entry Requirements: Contact the institution for details.

G50 THE UNIVERSITY OF GLOUCESTERSHIRE

HARDWICK CAMPUS
ST PAUL'S ROAD
CHELTENHAM GL50 4BS
t: 01242 714501 **f:** 01242 543334
e: admissions@glos.ac.uk
// www.glos.ac.uk

XC16 BSc Sports Coaching and Sports Development

Duration: 3FT Hon

Entry Requirements: *GCE:* 240-280.

CX61 BSc Sports Coaching and Sports Strength & Conditioning

Duration: 3FT Hon

Entry Requirements: *GCE:* 200-300.

G53 GLYNDWR UNIVERSITY

PLAS COCH
MOLD ROAD
WREXHAM LL11 2AW
t: 01978 293439 **f:** 01978 290008
e: SID@glyndwr.ac.uk
// www.glyndwr.ac.uk

C610 BSc Sports Coaching

Duration: 3FT Hon

Entry Requirements: *GCE:* 200.

G80 GRIMSBY INSTITUTE OF FURTHER AND HIGHER EDUCATION

NUNS CORNER
GRIMSBY
NE LINCOLNSHIRE DN34 5BQ
t: 0800 328 3631 **f:** 01472 315506/879924
e: headmissions@grimsby.ac.uk
// www.grimsby.ac.uk

CX61 FdA Sport Coaching

Duration: 2FT Fdg

Entry Requirements: HND required.

H49 UHI MILLENNIUM INSTITUTE

UHI EXECUTIVE OFFICE
NESS WALK
INVERNESS
SCOTLAND IV3 5SQ
t: 01463 279000 **f:** 01463 279001
e: info@uhi.ac.uk
// www.uhi.ac.uk

1X6C HND Sports Coaching with Development of Sport

Duration: 2FT HND

Entry Requirements: *SQAH:* C.

16XC HNC Sports Coaching with Development of Sport

Duration: 1FT HNC

Entry Requirements: *SQAH:* C.

H60 THE UNIVERSITY OF HUDDERSFIELD
QUEENSGATE
HUDDERSFIELD HD1 3DH

t: 01484 473969 **f:** 01484 472765
e: admissionsandrecords@hud.ac.uk

// www.hud.ac.uk

CX61 BSc Sports Coaching
Duration: 1FT Hon

Entry Requirements: *GCE:* 120. *SQAH:* CCC. *IB:* 24.

H72 THE UNIVERSITY OF HULL
THE UNIVERSITY OF HULL
COTTINGHAM ROAD
HULL HU6 7RX

t: 01482 466100 **f:** 01482 442290
e: admissions@hull.ac.uk

// www.hull.ac.uk

CB69 BSc Sports Coaching and Performance
Duration: 3FT Hon

Entry Requirements: *GCE:* 240-280. *IB:* 30.

K84 KINGSTON UNIVERSITY
STUDENT INFORMATION & ADVICE CENTRE
COOPER HOUSE
40-46 SURBITON ROAD
KINGSTON UPON THAMES KT1 2HX

t: 020 8547 7053 **f:** 020 8547 7080
e: aps@kingston.ac.uk

// www.kingston.ac.uk

CX6D BSc Sports Analysis & Coaching (including foundation)
Duration: 4FT Hon

Entry Requirements: *GCE:* 40.

CXP1 BSc Sports Analysis & Coaching (International only)
Duration: 4FT Hon

Entry Requirements: *GCE:* 40.

K90 KIRKLEES COLLEGE
HALIFAX ROAD
DEWSBURY
WEST YORKSHIRE WF13 2AS

t: 01924 436221 **f:** 01924 457047

CX61 FdSc Sports Coaching
Duration: 2FT Fdg

Entry Requirements: Contact the institution for details.

L27 LEEDS METROPOLITAN UNIVERSITY
COURSE ENQUIRIES OFFICE
CIVIC QUARTER
LEEDS LS1 3HE

t: 0113 81 23113 **f:** 0113 81 23129
e: course-enquiries@leedsmet.ac.uk

// www.leedsmet.ac.uk

CX6D BA/BSc Sports Coaching
Duration: 3FT Hon

Entry Requirements: Contact the institution for details.

CXQ1 FdSc Sports Performance
Duration: 2FT Hon

Entry Requirements: Contact the institution for details.

L53 COLEG LLANDRILLO CYMRU
LLANDUDNO ROAD
RHOS-ON-SEA
COLWYN BAY
NORTH WALES LL28 4HZ

t: 01492 542338/339 **f:** 01492 543052
e: degrees@llandrillo.ac.uk

// www.llandrillo.ac.uk

CX61 BSc Sports Coaching and Exercise Science
Duration: 1FT Hon

Entry Requirements: Interview required.

CX6C FdSc Sports Coaching and Exercise Science
Duration: 2FT Fdg

Entry Requirements: *GCE:* 160. *IB:* 24. Interview required.

M10 THE MANCHESTER COLLEGE
OPENSHAW CAMPUS
ASHTON OLD ROAD
OPENSHAW
MANCHESTER M11 2WH

t: 0800 068 8585 **f:** 0161 920 4103
e: enquiries@themanchestercollege.ac.uk

// www.themanchestercollege.ac.uk

CX61 FdA Sports Coaching
Duration: 2FT Fdg

Entry Requirements: *GCE:* 60.

M40 THE MANCHESTER METROPOLITAN UNIVERSITY

ADMISSIONS OFFICE
ALL SAINTS (GMS)
ALL SAINTS
MANCHESTER M15 6BH

t: 0161 247 2000

// www.mmu.ac.uk

LC5Q BA Abuse Studies/Coaching Studies

Duration: 3FT Hon

Entry Requirements: *BTEC ND:* MMM.

C611 BA Coaching and Sport Development (Foundation)

Duration: 4FT Hon

Entry Requirements: *GCE:* 80-120.

LC3Q BA Coaching Studies/Crime Studies

Duration: 3FT Hon

Entry Requirements: *BTEC ND:* MMM.

LCH6 BA Coaching Studies/Cultural Studies

Duration: 3FT Hon

Entry Requirements: *BTEC ND:* MMM.

CW6M BA Coaching Studies/Dance

Duration: 3FT Hon

Entry Requirements: *GCE:* 260. *BTEC ND:* DMM.

CXQ3 BA Coaching Studies/Education Studies

Duration: 3FT Hon

Entry Requirements: *BTEC ND:* MMM.

CB6Y BA Coaching Studies/Health Studies

Duration: 3FT Hon

Entry Requirements: *BTEC ND:* MMM.

CWQ3 BA Coaching Studies/Music

Duration: 3FT Hon

Entry Requirements: *GCE:* 260. *BTEC ND:* DMM.

WC36 BA Coaching Studies/Popular Music

Duration: 3FT Hon

Entry Requirements: *GCE:* 260. *BTEC ND:* DMM.

CX61 BSc Coaching Studies/Exercise & Physical Activity

Duration: 3FT Hon

Entry Requirements: *BTEC ND:* MMM.

CC6W BSc Coaching Studies/Psychology

Duration: 3FT Hon

Entry Requirements: *BTEC ND:* MMM.

M80 MIDDLESEX UNIVERSITY

MIDDLESEX UNIVERSITY
THE BURROUGHS
LONDON NW4 4BT

t: 020 8411 5555 **f:** 020 8411 5649
e: enquiries@mdx.ac.uk

// www.mdx.ac.uk

C600 FdSc Coaching and Sports Development

Duration: 2FT Fdg

Entry Requirements: Contact the institution for details.

M99 MYERSCOUGH COLLEGE

MYERSCOUGH HALL
BILSBORROW
PRESTON PR3 0RY

t: 01995 642222 **f:** 01995 642333
e: enquiries@myerscough.ac.uk

// www.myerscough.ac.uk

XC1P FdA Cricket Coaching and Development

Duration: 2FT Fdg

Entry Requirements: *GCE:* A-C. *SQAH:* AA-CC. *SQAAH:* A-C. *IB:* 24. *BTEC NC:* PP. *BTEC ND:* PPP.

CX6C FdA Football Coaching

Duration: 2FT Fdg

Entry Requirements: *GCE:* A-C. *SQAH:* AA-CC. *SQAAH:* A-C. *IB:* 24. *BTEC NC:* PP. *BTEC ND:* PPP.

C601 FdSc Golf Performance

Duration: 2FT Fdg

Entry Requirements: *GCE:* A-C. *SQAH:* AA-CC. *SQAAH:* A-C. *IB:* 24. *BTEC NC:* PP. *BTEC ND:* PPP.

C602 FdA Health and Personal Training

Duration: 2FT Fdg

Entry Requirements: *GCE:* A-C. *SQAH:* AA-CC. *SQAAH:* A-C. *IB:* 24. *BTEC NC:* PP. *BTEC ND:* PPP.

CX6D FdA Sports Coaching (Rugby)

Duration: 2FT Fdg

Entry Requirements: Contact the institution for details.

N13 NEATH PORT TALBOT COLLEGE

NEATH CAMPUS
DWR-Y-FELIN ROAD
NEATH
NEATH PORT TALBOT BOROUGH SA10 7RF

t: 01639 648033 f: 01639 648009
e: admissions@nptc.ac.uk

// www.nptc.ac.uk

CX61 FdA Coaching and Performance

Duration: 2FT Fdg

Entry Requirements: Contact the institution for details.

N23 NEWCASTLE COLLEGE

STUDENT SERVICES
RYE HILL CAMPUS
SCOTSWOOD ROAD
NEWCASTLE UPON TYNE NE4 7SA

t: 0191 200 4000 f: 0191 200 4349
e: enquiries@ncl-coll.ac.uk

// www.newcastlecollege.co.uk

CB69 FdSc Sports Training and Rehabilitation

Duration: 2FT Fdg

Entry Requirements: *GCE:* 120. *BTEC NC:* MP. *BTEC ND:* PPP.

N37 UNIVERSITY OF WALES, NEWPORT

CAERLEON CAMPUS
PO BOX 101
NEWPORT
SOUTH WALES NP18 3YH

t: 01633 432030 f: 01633 432850
e: admissions@newport.ac.uk

// www.newport.ac.uk

CX61 BSc Sports Coaching & Development

Duration: 3FT Hon

Entry Requirements: *GCE:* 240. *IB:* 24. Interview required.

N38 UNIVERSITY OF NORTHAMPTON

PARK CAMPUS
BOUGHTON GREEN ROAD
NORTHAMPTON NN2 7AL

t: 0800 358 2232 f: 01604 722083
e: admissions@northampton.ac.uk

// www.northampton.ac.uk

CX6C BSc Sports Performance and Coaching (top-up)

Duration: 1FT Hon

Entry Requirements: Contact the institution for details.

N49 NESCOT, SURREY

REIGATE ROAD
EWELL
EPSOM
SURREY KT17 3DS

t: 020 8394 3038 f: 020 8394 3030
e: info@nescot.ac.uk

// www.nescot.ac.uk

16XC HNC Sport and Exercise Science (Coaching & Teaching)

Duration: 1FT HNC

Entry Requirements: *GCE:* DD. *BTEC ND:* PPP.

N77 NORTHUMBRIA UNIVERSITY

TRINITY BUILDING
NORTHUMBERLAND ROAD
NEWCASTLE UPON TYNE NE1 8ST

t: 0191 243 7420 f: 0191 227 4561
e: er.admissions@northumbria.ac.uk

// www.northumbria.ac.uk

C6X1 BA Sport Development with Coaching

Duration: 3FT Hon

Entry Requirements: *GCE:* 280. *SQAH:* BBCCC. *SQAAH:* BCC. *IB:* 25. *BTEC ND:* DMM. *OCR ND:* Merit. *OCR NED:* Merit.

C6XC BSc Applied Sport Science with Coaching

Duration: 3FT Hon

Entry Requirements: *GCE:* 280. *SQAH:* BBCCC. *SQAAH:* BCC. *IB:* 25. *BTEC ND:* DMM. *OCR ND:* Merit. *OCR NED:* Merit.

O66 OXFORD BROOKES UNIVERSITY

ADMISSIONS OFFICE
HEADINGTON CAMPUS
GIPSY LANE
OXFORD OX3 0BP

t: 01865 483040 f: 01865 483983
e: admissions@brookes.ac.uk

// www.brookes.ac.uk

NC26 BA/BSc Business Management/Sports & Coaching Studies

Duration: 3FT Hon

Entry Requirements: *GCE:* BBC.

CXQ3 BA/BSc Early Childhood Studies/Sports and Coaching Studies

Duration: 3FT Hon

Entry Requirements: *GCE:* BCC.

CL67 BA/BSc Geography/Sports and Coaching Studies

Duration: 3FT Hon

Entry Requirements: *GCE:* BCC.

CV61 BA/BSc History/Sports and Coaching Studies

Duration: 3FT Hon

Entry Requirements: *GCE:* BBC.

CCP1 BSc/BA Biology/Sports and Coaching Studies

Duration: 3FT Hon

Entry Requirements: *GCE:* BBB.

P60 UNIVERSITY OF PLYMOUTH

DRAKE CIRCUS
PLYMOUTH PL4 8AA

t: 01752 588037 **f:** 01752 588050
e: admissions@plymouth.ac.uk

// www.plymouth.ac.uk

C609 FdSc Strength Conditioning and Sports Coaching

Duration: 2FT Fdg

Entry Requirements: Interview required.

P63 UCP MARJON - UNIVERSITY COLLEGE PLYMOUTH ST MARK & ST JOHN

DERRIFORD ROAD
PLYMOUTH PL6 8BH

t: 01752 636890 **f:** 01752 636819
e: admissions@marjon.ac.uk

// www.ucpmarjon.ac.uk

X151 BA Coach and Physical Education

Duration: 3FT Hon

Entry Requirements: *GCE:* 240.

CX63 BSc Coach & Fitness Education

Duration: 1FT Hon

Entry Requirements: Contact the institution for details.

CX6C FdA Sports Development and Coaching

Duration: 2FT Fdg

Entry Requirements: *GCE:* 40.

R48 ROEHAMPTON UNIVERSITY

ERASMUS HOUSE
ROEHAMPTON LANE
LONDON SW15 5PU

t: 020 8392 3232 **f:** 020 8392 3470
e: enquiries@roehampton.ac.uk

// www.roehampton.ac.uk

XC16 FdA Sports Coaching Practice

Duration: 2FT Fdg

Entry Requirements: Contact the institution for details.

S26 SOLIHULL COLLEGE

BLOSSOMFIELD ROAD
SOLIHULL
WEST MIDLANDS B91 1SB

t: 0121 678 7247 **f:** 0121 678 7200
e: enquiries@solihull.ac.uk

// www.solihull.ac.uk

CX61 FdA Sports Coaching

Duration: 2FT Fdg

Entry Requirements: Contact the institution for details.

S30 SOUTHAMPTON SOLENT UNIVERSITY

EAST PARK TERRACE
SOUTHAMPTON
HAMPSHIRE SO14 0RT

t: +44 (0) 23 8031 9039 **f:** + 44 (0)23 8022 2259
e: admissions@solent.ac.uk or ask@solent.ac.uk

// www.solent.ac.uk/

CX6D BSc Sport Coaching

Duration: 3FT Hon

Entry Requirements: *GCE:* 240.

S46 SOUTH NOTTINGHAM COLLEGE

WEST BRIDGFORD CENTRE
GREYTHORN DRIVE
WEST BRIDGFORD
NOTTINGHAM NG2 7GA

t: 0115 914 6400 **f:** 0115 914 6444
e: enquiries@south-nottingham.ac.uk

// www.snc.ac.uk

CX69 FdSc Applied Sport Coaching

Duration: 2FT Fdg

Entry Requirements: *GCE:* 80. *BTEC NC:* PP. *BTEC ND:* PPP.

S64 ST MARY'S UNIVERSITY COLLEGE, TWICKENHAM

WALDEGRAVE ROAD
STRAWBERRY HILL
MIDDLESEX TW1 4SX

t: 020 8240 4029 f: 020 8240 2361
e: admit@smuc.ac.uk

// www.smuc.ac.uk

CN6F BA/BSc Coaching Science and Management Studies
Duration: 3FT Hon

Entry Requirements: *GCE:* 160-200. *BTEC NC:* MM. *BTEC ND:* MPP.

C601 BSc Coaching Science
Duration: 3FT Hon

Entry Requirements: *GCE:* 160-200. *BTEC NC:* MM. *BTEC ND:* MPP.

S72 STAFFORDSHIRE UNIVERSITY

COLLEGE ROAD
STOKE ON TRENT ST4 2DE

t: 01782 292753 f: 01782 292740
e: admissions@staffs.ac.uk

// www.staffs.ac.uk

C603 BA Sports Development and Coaching
Duration: 3FT Hon

Entry Requirements: *GCE:* 180-240. *IB:* 24. *BTEC NC:* DM. *BTEC ND:* MMM.

S73 STAFFORDSHIRE UNIVERSITY REGIONAL FEDERATION

COLLEGE ROAD
STOKE ON TRENT ST4 2DE

t: 01782 292753 f: 01782 292740
e: admissions@staffs.ac.uk

// www.surf.ac.uk

CX63 BA Sports Development & Coaching
Duration: 4FT Hon

Entry Requirements: *GCE:* 80-120.

106C HND Sports Performance and Coaching
Duration: 2FT HND

Entry Requirements: *GCE:* 40-80. *IB:* 24.

S82 UNIVERSITY CAMPUS SUFFOLK

WATERFRONT BUILDING
NEPTUNE QUAY
IPSWICH
SUFFOLK IP4 1QJ

t: 01473 338348 f: 01473 339900
e: info@ucs.ac.uk

// www.ucs.ac.uk

C6BX BA Personal Training with Sports Therapy (Level 3 entry only)
Duration: 1FT Hon

Entry Requirements: Contact the institution for details.

C6B9 FdA Personal Training with Sports Therapy
Duration: 2FT Fdg

Entry Requirements: *GCE:* 200.

S84 UNIVERSITY OF SUNDERLAND

STUDENT HELPLINE
THE STUDENT GATEWAY
CHESTER ROAD
SUNDERLAND SR1 3SD

t: 0191 515 3000 f: 0191 515 3805
e: student-helpline@sunderland.ac.uk

// www.sunderland.ac.uk

CX6C BSc Sports Coaching
Duration: 3FT Hon

Entry Requirements: *GCE:* 240-360. *IB:* 36. *BTEC NC:* DD. *BTEC ND:* MMM. *OCR ND:* Distinction. *OCR NED:* Merit.

CX6D FdSc Sports Coaching
Duration: 2FT Fdg

Entry Requirements: *GCE:* 100-240. *BTEC NC:* MP. *BTEC ND:* PPP. *OCR ND:* Pass. *OCR NED:* Pass.

T20 UNIVERSITY OF TEESSIDE

MIDDLESBROUGH TS1 3BA

t: 01642 218121 f: 01642 384201
e: registry@tees.ac.uk

// www.tees.ac.uk

C603 FdSc Fitness Instruction and Sports Massage
Duration: 2FT Fdg

Entry Requirements: *GCE:* 120.

T85 TRURO AND PENWITH COLLEGE (FORMERLY TRURO COLLEGE)

TRURO COLLEGE
COLLEGE ROAD
TRURO
CORNWALL TR1 3XX

t: 01872 267122 f: 01872 267526
e: heinfo@trurocollege.ac.uk

// www.trurocollege.ac.uk

C601 BSc (Hons) Sports Performance and Coaching

Duration: 1FT Deg

Entry Requirements: Contact the institution for details.

C600 FdSc Personal Trainer

Duration: 2FT Fdg

Entry Requirements: *GCE:* 60. *IB:* 24. *BTEC NC:* PP. *BTEC ND:* PPP.

C603 FdSc Sports Coaching & Therapy

Duration: 2FT Fdg

Entry Requirements: *GCE:* 60-80. *IB:* 24. *BTEC NC:* PP. *BTEC ND:* PPP.

U40 UNIVERSITY OF THE WEST OF SCOTLAND

PAISLEY
RENFREWSHIRE
SCOTLAND PA1 2BE

t: 0141 848 3727 f: 0141 848 3623
e: admissions@uws.ac.uk

// www.uws.ac.uk

CX61 DipHE Sport Coaching

Duration: 2FT Dip

Entry Requirements: *SQAH:* CC.

W08 WAKEFIELD COLLEGE

MARGARET STREET
WAKEFIELD
WEST YORKSHIRE WF1 2DH

t: 01924 789111 f: 01924 789281
e: courseinfo@wakefield.ac.uk

// www.wakefield.ac.uk

CX6D BSc Sports Performance Coaching

Duration: 1FT Hon

Entry Requirements: Contact the institution for details.

W25 WARWICKSHIRE COLLEGE

WARWICK NEW ROAD
LEAMINGTON SPA
WARWICKSHIRE CV32 5JE

t: 01926 318 000 f: 01926 318 111
e: he@warkscol.ac.uk

// www.warkscol.ac.uk

CX61 BSc Performance Coaching(Pathways in Tennis and Football)

Duration: 3FT Hon

Entry Requirements: Contact the institution for details.

W67 WIGAN AND LEIGH COLLEGE

PO BOX 53
PARSONS WALK
WIGAN WN1 1RS

t: 01942 761605 f: 01942 760223

// www.wigan-leigh.ac.uk

BC96 FdA Health & Personal Trainer

Duration: 2FT Fdg

Entry Requirements: Contact the institution for details.

CX61 FdSc Sports Coaching

Duration: 2FT Fdg

Entry Requirements: *GCE:* D. *BTEC NC:* PP. *BTEC ND:* PPP. Interview required.

W76 UNIVERSITY OF WINCHESTER

WINCHESTER
HANTS SO22 4NR

t: 01962 827234 f: 01962 827288
e: course.enquiries@winchester.ac.uk

// www.winchester.ac.uk

CX61 BA Sports Coaching and Development

Duration: 3FT Hon

Entry Requirements: *Foundation:* Distinction. *GCE:* 240-280. *IB:* 24. *BTEC NC:* DD. *BTEC ND:* MMM. *OCR ND:* Distinction.

CX6C DipHE Sports Coaching and Development

Duration: 2FT Dip

Entry Requirements: *Foundation:* Pass. *GCE:* 120. *IB:* 20. *BTEC NC:* MP. *BTEC ND:* PPP.

W80 UNIVERSITY OF WORCESTER

HENWICK GROVE
WORCESTER WR2 6AJ

t: 01905 855111 **f:** 01905 855377
e: admissions@worc.ac.uk

// www.worcester.ac.uk

XCH6 BA Education Studies and Sports Coaching Science

Duration: 3FT Hon

Entry Requirements: *GCE:* 240. *IB:* 24. *BTEC NC:* DD. *BTEC ND:* MMM. *OCR ND:* Distinction. *OCR NED:* Merit.

TC76 BA/BSc American Studies and Sports Coaching Science

Duration: 3FT Hon

Entry Requirements: *GCE:* 240-260. *IB:* 24. *BTEC NC:* DD. *BTEC ND:* MMM. *OCR ND:* Distinction. *OCR NED:* Merit.

NCF6 BA/BSc Business Management and Sports Coaching Science

Duration: 3FT Hon

Entry Requirements: *GCE:* 240. *IB:* 24. *BTEC NC:* DD. *BTEC ND:* MMM. *OCR ND:* Distinction. *OCR NED:* Merit.

QCH6 BA/BSc English Literary Studies and Sports Coaching Science

Duration: 3FT Hon

Entry Requirements: *GCE:* 240-260. *IB:* 24. *BTEC NC:* DD. *BTEC ND:* MMM. *OCR ND:* Distinction. *OCR NED:* Merit.

CL67 BA/BSc Human Geography and Sports Coaching Science

Duration: 3FT Hon

Entry Requirements: *GCE:* 240-260. *IB:* 24. *BTEC NC:* DD. *BTEC ND:* MMM. *OCR ND:* Distinction. *OCR NED:* Merit.

DC36 BSc Animal Biology and Sports Coaching Science

Duration: 3FT Hon

Entry Requirements: *GCE:* 240. *IB:* 24. *BTEC ND:* DMM. *OCR ND:* Distinction. *OCR NED:* Merit.

CC16 BSc Biology and Sports Coaching Science

Duration: 3FT Hon

Entry Requirements: *GCE:* 240. *IB:* 24. *BTEC ND:* DMM. *OCR ND:* Distinction. *OCR NED:* Merit.

GC46 BSc Computing and Sports Coaching Science

Duration: 3FT Hon

Entry Requirements: *GCE:* 240. *IB:* 24. *BTEC NC:* DD. *BTEC ND:* MMM. *OCR ND:* Distinction. *OCR NED:* Merit.

GC4P BSc Computing and Sports Studies

Duration: 3FT Hon

Entry Requirements: *GCE:* 240. *IB:* 24. *BTEC NC:* DD. *BTEC ND:* MMM. *OCR ND:* Distinction. *OCR NED:* Merit.

LCR6 BSc Geography and Sports Coaching Science

Duration: 3FT Hon

Entry Requirements: *GCE:* 240-260. *IB:* 24. *BTEC NC:* DD. *BTEC ND:* MMM. *OCR ND:* Distinction. *OCR NED:* Merit.

CC61 BSc Human Biology and Sports Coaching Science

Duration: 3FT Hon

Entry Requirements: *GCE:* 240. *IB:* 24. *BTEC ND:* DMM. *OCR ND:* Distinction. *OCR NED:* Merit.

BC46 BSc Human Nutrition and Sports Coaching Science

Duration: 3FT Hon

Entry Requirements: *GCE:* 240. *IB:* 24. *BTEC ND:* DMM. *OCR ND:* Distinction. *OCR NED:* Merit.

C690 BSc Physical Education and Sports Coaching Science

Duration: 3FT Hon

Entry Requirements: *GCE:* 240. *IB:* 24. *BTEC NC:* DD. *BTEC ND:* MMM. *OCR ND:* Distinction. *OCR NED:* Merit.

CF68 BSc Physical Geography and Sports Coaching Science

Duration: 3FT Hon

Entry Requirements: *GCE:* 240-260. *IB:* 24. *BTEC NC:* DD. *BTEC ND:* MMM. *OCR ND:* Distinction. *OCR NED:* Merit.

C601 BSc Sports Coaching Science

Duration: 3FT Hon

Entry Requirements: *GCE:* 240. *IB:* 24. *BTEC NC:* DD. *BTEC ND:* MMM. *OCR ND:* Distinction. *OCR NED:* Merit.

26NC HND Sports Coaching and Management

Duration: 2FT HND

Entry Requirements: *GCE:* 120. *IB:* 24. *BTEC NC:* MP. *BTEC ND:* PPP. *OCR ND:* Merit. *OCR NED:* Pass.

16XC HND Sports Performance and Coaching
Duration: 2FT HND

Entry Requirements: *GCE:* 120. *IB:* 24. *BTEC NC:* MP. *BTEC ND:* PPP. *OCR ND:* Merit. *OCR NED:* Pass.

Y75 YORK ST JOHN UNIVERSITY
LORD MAYOR'S WALK
YORK YO31 7EX

t: 01904 876598 f: 01904 876940/876921
e: admissions@yorksj.ac.uk

// www.yorksj.ac.uk

CB69 BSc Exercise Instruction & Referral
Duration: 3FT Hon

Entry Requirements: Contact the institution for details.

C602 BSc Sport Performance Conditioning
Duration: 3FT Hon

Entry Requirements: Contact the institution for details.

PHYSIOTHERAPY

B32 THE UNIVERSITY OF BIRMINGHAM
EDGBASTON
BIRMINGHAM B15 2TT

t: 0121 415 8900 f: 0121 414 7159
e: admissions@bham.ac.uk

// www.bham.ac.uk

B160 BSc Physiotherapy (including state registration)
Duration: 3FT Hon

Entry Requirements: *GCE:* ABB. *SQAH:* AAAAA-ABBBB. *SQAAH:* ABB. *IB:* 34. *BTEC ND:* DDM. Interview required.

B50 BOURNEMOUTH UNIVERSITY
TALBOT CAMPUS
FERN BARROW
POOLE
DORSET BH12 5BB

t: 01202 524111

// www.bournemouth.ac.uk

B160 BSc Physiotherapy
Duration: 3FT Hon

Entry Requirements: *GCE:* 320.

B56 THE UNIVERSITY OF BRADFORD
RICHMOND ROAD
BRADFORD
WEST YORKSHIRE BD7 1DP

t: 0800 073 1225 f: 01274 235585
e: course-enquiries@bradford.ac.uk

// www.bradford.ac.uk

B160 BSc Physiotherapy
Duration: 3FT Hon

Entry Requirements: *GCE:* BBB. *IB:* 32. *BTEC NC:* DM. *BTEC ND:* DMM. Interview required.

B80 UNIVERSITY OF THE WEST OF ENGLAND, BRISTOL
FRENCHAY CAMPUS
COLDHARBOUR LANE
BRISTOL BS16 1QY

t: +44 (0)117 32 83333 f: +44 (0)117 32 82810
e: admissions@uwe.ac.uk

// www.uwe.ac.uk

B160 BSc Physiotherapy
Duration: 3FT Hon

Entry Requirements: *GCE:* 280-340.

B84 BRUNEL UNIVERSITY
UXBRIDGE
MIDDLESEX UB8 3PH

t: 01895 265265 f: 01895 269790
e: admissions@brunel.ac.uk

// www.brunel.ac.uk

B160 BSc Physiotherapy
Duration: 3FT Hon

Entry Requirements: *GCE:* 320. *IB:* 31. *BTEC ND:* DDM.

C15 CARDIFF UNIVERSITY
PO BOX 927
30-36 NEWPORT ROAD
CARDIFF CF24 0DE

t: 029 2087 9999 f: 029 2087 6138
e: admissions@cardiff.ac.uk

// www.cardiff.ac.uk

B160 BSc Physiotherapy
Duration: 3FT Hon

Entry Requirements: *GCE:* AAB. *SQAAH:* AAB. *IB:* 27. *BTEC NC:* DD. *BTEC ND:* DDD.

C30 UNIVERSITY OF CENTRAL LANCASHIRE

PRESTON
LANCS PR1 2HE

t: 01772 201201 f: 01772 894954
e: uadmissions@uclan.ac.uk
// www.uclan.ac.uk

B160 BSc Physiotherapy

Duration: 3FT Hon

Entry Requirements: *GCE:* BBB. *IB:* 32. *BTEC NC:* DD. *BTEC ND:*
DDM. Interview required.

C85 COVENTRY UNIVERSITY

THE STUDENT CENTRE
COVENTRY UNIVERSITY
1 GULSON RD
COVENTRY CV1 2JH

t: 024 7615 2222 f: 024 7615 2223
e: studentenquiries@coventry.ac.uk
// www.coventry.ac.uk

B160 BSc Physiotherapy

Duration: 3FT Hon

Entry Requirements: *GCE:* 350. *BTEC ND:* DDD.

E28 UNIVERSITY OF EAST LONDON

DOCKLANDS CAMPUS
UNIVERSITY WAY
LONDON E16 2RD

t: 020 8223 2835 f: 020 8223 2978
e: admiss@uel.ac.uk
// www.uel.ac.uk

B160 BSc Physiotherapy

Duration: 3FT Hon

Entry Requirements: *GCE:* 300. *IB:* 30.

B161 BSc Physiotherapy (by situated learning)

Duration: 3FT Hon

Entry Requirements: *GCE:* 280.

H36 UNIVERSITY OF HERTFORDSHIRE

UNIVERSITY ADMISSIONS SERVICE
COLLEGE LANE
HATFIELD
HERTS AL10 9AB

t: 01707 284800 f: 01707 284870
// www.herts.ac.uk

B160 BSc Physiotherapy

Duration: 3FT Hon

Entry Requirements: *GCE:* 300.

K12 KEELE UNIVERSITY

STAFFS ST5 5BG

t: 01782 734005 f: 01782 632343
e: undergraduate@keele.ac.uk
// www.keele.ac.uk

B160 BSc Physiotherapy

Duration: 3FT Hon

Entry Requirements: *GCE:* BBB. *SQAAH:* BBB. *IB:* 28. *BTEC ND:*
DDM. Interview required.

B1B9 BSc Physiotherapy with Health Foundation Year

Duration: 4FT Hon

Entry Requirements: *GCE:* BBB. *SQAAH:* BBB. *IB:* 28. *BTEC ND:*
DDM. Interview required.

K60 KING'S COLLEGE LONDON (UNIVERSITY OF LONDON)

STRAND
LONDON WC2R 2LS

t: 020 7836 5454 f: 020 7836 1799
e: ucas.enquiries@kcl.ac.uk
// www.kcl.ac.uk

B160 BSc Physiotherapy

Duration: 3FT Hon

Entry Requirements: *GCE:* BBB. *SQAH:* ABBBB. *IB:* 32.

L39 UNIVERSITY OF LINCOLN

ADMISSIONS
BRAYFORD POOL
LINCOLN LN6 7TS

t: 01522 886097 f: 01522 886146
e: admissions@lincoln.ac.uk
// www.lincoln.ac.uk

B160 CertHE Health Science (Physiotherapy)

Duration: 1FT Cer

Entry Requirements: Interview required.

L41 THE UNIVERSITY OF LIVERPOOL

THE FOUNDATION BUILDING
BROWNLOW HILL
LIVERPOOL L69 7ZX

t: 0151 794 2000 f: 0151 708 6502
e: ugrecruitment@liv.ac.uk
// www.liv.ac.uk

B160 BSc Physiotherapy

Duration: 3FT Hon

Entry Requirements: *GCE:* BBB. *SQAH:* BBBBB. *SQAAH:* BBB. *IB:* 30.
BTEC ND: DDM. Interview required.

L46 LIVERPOOL HOPE UNIVERSITY

HOPE PARK
LIVERPOOL L16 9JD

t: 0151 291 3295 **f:** 0151 291 2050
e: admission@hope.ac.uk

// www.hope.ac.uk

XC11 BA Disability Studies and Environmental Biology

Duration: 3FT Hon

Entry Requirements: *GCE:* 240. *IB:* 25.

M40 THE MANCHESTER METROPOLITAN UNIVERSITY

ADMISSIONS OFFICE
ALL SAINTS (GMS)
ALL SAINTS
MANCHESTER M15 6BH

t: 0161 247 2000

// www.mmu.ac.uk

B160 BSc Physiotherapy

Duration: 3FT Hon

Entry Requirements: *GCE:* BBB. *SQAH:* AABBB. *SQAAH:* B. *IB:* 30.
BTEC ND: DDM. Interview required.

O66 OXFORD BROOKES UNIVERSITY

ADMISSIONS OFFICE
HEADINGTON CAMPUS
GIPSY LANE
OXFORD OX3 0BP

t: 01865 483040 **f:** 01865 483983
e: admissions@brookes.ac.uk

// www.brookes.ac.uk

B160 BSc Physiotherapy

Duration: 3FT Hon

Entry Requirements: *GCE:* BBB. *SQAAH:* BBB.

P60 UNIVERSITY OF PLYMOUTH

DRAKE CIRCUS
PLYMOUTH PL4 8AA

t: 01752 588037 **f:** 01752 588050
e: admissions@plymouth.ac.uk

// www.plymouth.ac.uk

B160 BSc Physiotherapy

Duration: 3FT Hon

Entry Requirements: *GCE:* 300. *IB:* 33. *BTEC NC:* DD. *BTEC ND:*
DDM. *OCR ND:* Distinction. *OCR NED:* Merit.

Q25 QUEEN MARGARET UNIVERSITY , EDINBURGH

QUEEN MARGARET UNIVERSITY DRIVE
EDINBURGH EH21 6UU

t: 0131474 0000 **f:** 0131 474 0001
e: admissions@qmu.ac.uk

// www.qmu.ac.uk

B160 BSc Physiotherapy

Duration: 4FT Hon

Entry Requirements: *GCE:* 320. *IB:* 30.

R36 THE ROBERT GORDON UNIVERSITY

ROBERT GORDON UNIVERSITY
SCHOOLHILL
ABERDEEN
SCOTLAND AB10 1FR

t: 01224 26 27 28 **f:** 01224 262147
e: admissions@rgu.ac.uk

// www.rgu.ac.uk

B160 BSc Physiotherapy

Duration: 4FT Hon

Entry Requirements: *GCE:* 300. *SQAH:* ABBC-BBBB. *IB:* 32. Interview
required.

S03 THE UNIVERSITY OF SALFORD

SALFORD M5 4WT

t: 0161 295 4545 **f:** 0161 295 3126
e: ugadmissions-exrel@salford.ac.uk

// www.salford.ac.uk

B160 BSc Physiotherapy

Duration: 3FT Hon

Entry Requirements: *GCE:* 300. *SQAH:* AABBB. *SQAAH:* BBB. *IB:* 32.
BTEC ND: DDM.

S21 SHEFFIELD HALLAM UNIVERSITY

CITY CAMPUS
HOWARD STREET
SHEFFIELD S1 1WB

t: 0114 225 5555 **f:** 0114 225 2167
e: admissions@shu.ac.uk

// www.shu.ac.uk

B160 BSc Physiotherapy

Duration: 3FT Hon

Entry Requirements: *GCE:* 300.

S27 UNIVERSITY OF SOUTHAMPTON

HIGHFIELD
SOUTHAMPTON SO17 1BJ

t: 023 8059 4732 f: 023 8059 3037
e: admissions@soton.ac.uk

// www.southampton.ac.uk

B160 BSc Physiotherapy

Duration: 3FT Hon

Entry Requirements: *GCE:* ABBb. *IB:* 33.

S49 ST GEORGE'S, UNIVERSITY OF LONDON

CRANMER TERRACE
LONDON SW17 0RE

t: +44 (0)20 8725 2333 f: +44 (0)20 8266 6282
e: enquiries@sgul.ac.uk

// www.sgul.ac.uk

B160 BSc Physiotherapy

Duration: 3FT Hon

Entry Requirements: *GCE:* 300. Interview required.

T20 UNIVERSITY OF TEESSIDE

MIDDLESBROUGH TS1 3BA

t: 01642 218121 f: 01642 384201
e: registry@tees.ac.uk

// www.tees.ac.uk

B160 BSc Physiotherapy

Duration: 3FT Hon

Entry Requirements: *GCE:* 300. *BTEC NC:* DM. *BTEC ND:* DDM.
Interview required.

U20 UNIVERSITY OF ULSTER

COLERAINE
CO. LONDONDERRY
NORTHERN IRELAND BT52 1SA

t: 028 7032 4221 f: 028 7032 4908
e: online@ulster.ac.uk

// www.ulster.ac.uk

B160 BSc Physiotherapy

Duration: 3FT Hon

Entry Requirements: *GCE:* BBB. *SQAH:* AABCC. *SQAAH:* BBB. *IB:* 25.
BTEC NC: DD. *BTEC ND:* DDD. Admissions Test required.

Y75 YORK ST JOHN UNIVERSITY

LORD MAYOR'S WALK
YORK YO31 7EX

t: 01904 876598 f: 01904 876940/876921
e: admissions@yorksj.ac.uk

// www.yorksj.ac.uk

B160 BSc Physiotherapy

Duration: 3FT Hon

Entry Requirements: *GCE:* 280. *SQAH:* BBBBBB-BBBCCC. *SQAAH:*
AAB-BBB. *IB:* 30. *OCR ND:* Distinction. Interview required.

PODIATRY

B72 UNIVERSITY OF BRIGHTON

MITHRAS HOUSE
LEWES ROAD
BRIGHTON BN2 4AT

t: 01273 644644 f: 01273 642607
e: admissions@brighton.ac.uk

// www.brighton.ac.uk

B985 BSc Podiatry

Duration: 3FT Hon

Entry Requirements: *GCE:* CCC. *IB:* 28. Interview required.

C20 UNIVERSITY OF WALES INSTITUTE, CARDIFF

PO BOX 377
LLANDAFF CAMPUS
WESTERN AVENUE
CARDIFF CF5 2SG

t: 029 2041 6070 f: 029 2041 6286
e: admissions@uwic.ac.uk

// www.uwic.ac.uk

B985 BSc Podiatry

Duration: 3FT Hon

Entry Requirements: *GCE:* 220. *IB:* 24. *BTEC NC:* DD. *BTEC ND:*
MMM. *OCR ND:* Distinction.

E28 UNIVERSITY OF EAST LONDON

DOCKLANDS CAMPUS
UNIVERSITY WAY
LONDON E16 2RD

t: 020 8223 2835 f: 020 8223 2978
e: admiss@uel.ac.uk

// www.uel.ac.uk

B330 BSc Podiatric Medicine

Duration: 3FT Hon

Entry Requirements: *GCE:* 240.

G42 GLASGOW CALEDONIAN UNIVERSITY

CITY CAMPUS
COWCADDENS ROAD
GLASGOW G4 0BA

t: 0141 331 3000 f: 0141 331 3449
e: admissions@gcal.ac.uk

// www.gcal.ac.uk

B985 BSc Podiatry

Duration: 4FT Hon

Entry Requirements: *GCE:* CC. *SQAH:* BBCC.

H60 THE UNIVERSITY OF HUDDERSFIELD

QUEENSGATE
HUDDERSFIELD HD1 3DH

t: 01484 473969 f: 01484 472765
e: admissionsandrecords@hud.ac.uk

// www.hud.ac.uk

B985 BSc Podiatry

Duration: 3FT Hon

Entry Requirements: *GCE:* 220. *SQAH:* BBBC. *IB:* 26. Interview required.

M60 MATTHEW BOULTON COLLEGE OF FURTHER AND HIGHER EDUCATION

JENNENS ROAD
BIRMINGHAM B4 7PS

t: 0121 446 4545 f: 0121 503 8590
e: ask@mbc.ac.uk

// www.mbc.ac.uk

B985 BSc Podiatry

Duration: 3FT Hon

Entry Requirements: *GCE:* 80-160.

N28 NEW COLLEGE DURHAM

FRAMWELLGATE MOOR CENTRE
DURHAM DH1 5ES

t: 0191 375 4210/4211 f: 0191 375 4222
e: admissions@newdur.ac.uk

// www.newdur.ac.uk

B988 BSc Podiatry (with foundation year and state registration)

Duration: 4FT Hon

Entry Requirements: Interview required.

B985 BSc Podiatry (with state registration)

Duration: 3FT Hon

Entry Requirements: *GCE:* 160. Interview required.

N38 UNIVERSITY OF NORTHAMPTON

PARK CAMPUS
BOUGHTON GREEN ROAD
NORTHAMPTON NN2 7AL

t: 0800 358 2232 f: 01604 722083
e: admissions@northampton.ac.uk

// www.northampton.ac.uk

B985 BSc Podiatry

Duration: 3FT Hon

Entry Requirements: *GCE:* 220-260. *SQAH:* AAB-BBBB. *IB:* 24.

P60 UNIVERSITY OF PLYMOUTH

DRAKE CIRCUS
PLYMOUTH PL4 8AA

t: 01752 588037 f: 01752 588050
e: admissions@plymouth.ac.uk

// www.plymouth.ac.uk

B985 BSc Podiatry

Duration: 3FT Hon

Entry Requirements: *GCE:* 240-260. *IB:* 27. *BTEC NC:* DD. *BTEC ND:* MMM. *OCR ND:* Distinction. *OCR NED:* Merit.

Q25 QUEEN MARGARET UNIVERSITY , EDINBURGH

QUEEN MARGARET UNIVERSITY DRIVE
EDINBURGH EH21 6UU

t: 0131474 0000 f: 0131 474 0001
e: admissions@qmu.ac.uk

// www.qmu.ac.uk

B985 BSc Podiatry

Duration: 4FT Hon

Entry Requirements: *GCE:* 160. *IB:* 26.

S03 THE UNIVERSITY OF SALFORD

SALFORD M5 4WT

t: 0161 295 4545 f: 0161 295 3126
e: ugadmissions-exrel@salford.ac.uk

// www.salford.ac.uk

B985 BSc Podiatry

Duration: 3FT Hon

Entry Requirements: *GCE:* 240. *SQAH:* BCCCC. *SQAAH:* CCC. *IB:* 24. *BTEC NC:* DD. *BTEC ND:* MMM.

S27 UNIVERSITY OF SOUTHAMPTON

HIGHFIELD
SOUTHAMPTON SO17 1BJ

t: 023 8059 4732 f: 023 8059 3037
e: admissions@soton.ac.uk

// www.southampton.ac.uk

B985 BSc Podiatry

Duration: 3FT Hon

Entry Requirements: *GCE:* BBB. *IB:* 28.

U20 UNIVERSITY OF ULSTER

COLERAINE
CO. LONDONDERRY
NORTHERN IRELAND BT52 1SA

t: 028 7032 4221 f: 028 7032 4908
e: online@ulster.ac.uk

// www.ulster.ac.uk

B985 BSc Podiatry

Duration: 3FT Hon

Entry Requirements: *GCE:* BBB. *SQAH:* AABCC. *SQAAH:* BBB. *IB:* 25. *BTEC NC:* MM. *BTEC ND:* DDM. Admissions Test required.

ANATOMY, MEDICAL BIOCHEMISTRY AND HUMAN PHYSIOLOGY

A20 THE UNIVERSITY OF ABERDEEN

UNIVERSITY OFFICE
KING'S COLLEGE
ABERDEEN AB24 3FX

t: +44 (0) 1224 273504 f: +44 (0) 1224 272034
e: sras@abdn.ac.uk

// www.abdn.ac.uk/sras

CX11 BSc Biology and Education

Duration: 4FT Hon

Entry Requirements: *GCE:* 240. *SQAH:* BBBB. *SQAAH:* BCC. *IB:* 28. *BTEC ND:* MMM.

A40 ABERYSTWYTH UNIVERSITY

WELCOME CENTRE, ABERYSTWYTH UNIVERSITY
PENGLAIS CAMPUS
ABERYSTWYTH
CEREDIGION SY23 3FB

t: 01970 622021 f: 01970 627410
e: ug-admissions@aber.ac.uk

// www.aber.ac.uk

CC16 BSc Biology and Sports Science

Duration: 3FT Hon

Entry Requirements: *GCE:* 240-280. *IB:* 26.

C30 UNIVERSITY OF CENTRAL LANCASHIRE

PRESTON
LANCS PR1 2HE

t: 01772 201201 f: 01772 894954
e: uadmissions@uclan.ac.uk

// www.uclan.ac.uk

CB61 BSc Sport & Exercise Physiology (Top-up)

Duration: 1FT Hon

Entry Requirements: HND required.

C55 UNIVERSITY OF CHESTER

PARKGATE ROAD
CHESTER CH1 4BJ

t: 01244 511000 f: 01244 511300
e: enquiries@chester.ac.uk

// www.chester.ac.uk

CC16 BSc Biology and Sport & Exercise Sciences

Duration: 3FT Hon

Entry Requirements: *GCE:* 240. *SQAH:* BBBB. *IB:* 24. *BTEC NC:* DM. *BTEC ND:* MMM.

C1C6 BSc Biology with Sport & Exercise Sciences

Duration: 3FT Hon

Entry Requirements: *GCE:* 240. *SQAH:* BBBB. *IB:* 24. *BTEC NC:* DM. *BTEC ND:* MMM.

D65 UNIVERSITY OF DUNDEE

DUNDEE DD1 4HN

t: 01382 383838 f: 01382 388150
e: srs@dundee.ac.uk

//www.dundee.ac.uk/admissions/undergraduate

B1C6 BSc Physiology with Sports Biomedicine

Duration: 4FT Hon

Entry Requirements: *GCE:* CCC. *SQAH:* BBBB. *IB:* 28. *BTEC ND:* MMM.

E59 EDINBURGH NAPIER UNIVERSITY

CRAIGLOCKHART CAMPUS
EDINBURGH EH14 1DJ

t: +44 (0)8452 60 60 40 f: 0131 455 6464
e: info@napier.ac.uk

// www.napier.ac.uk

CB61 BSc Sport and Exercise Science (Exercise Physiology)

Duration: 3FT/4FT Ord/Hon

Entry Requirements: *GCE:* 260.

G28 UNIVERSITY OF GLASGOW

THE UNIVERSITY OF GLASGOW
THE FRASER BUILDING
65 HILLHEAD STREET
GLASGOW G12 8QF

t: 0141 330 6062 **f:** 0141 330 2961
e: ugenquiries@gla.ac.uk (UK/EU undergrad enquiries only)

// www.glasgow.ac.uk

C741 BSc Medical Biochemistry (Faster Route)

Duration: 3FT Hon

Entry Requirements: *GCE:* AAB. *SQAAH:* AAB.

BC16 BSc Physiology and Sports Science

Duration: 4FT Hon

Entry Requirements: *GCE:* BBB. *SQAH:* BBBB. *IB:* 30.

C743 MSci Medical Biochemistry with Work Placement (Faster Route)

Duration: 4FT Hon

Entry Requirements: *GCE:* AAB. *SQAAH:* AAB.

H36 UNIVERSITY OF HERTFORDSHIRE

UNIVERSITY ADMISSIONS SERVICE
COLLEGE LANE
HATFIELD
HERTS AL10 9AB

t: 01707 284800 **f:** 01707 284870

// www.herts.ac.uk

C6B1 BSc Sports Studies/Human Biology

Duration: 3FT/4SW Hon

Entry Requirements: *GCE:* 260.

H60 THE UNIVERSITY OF HUDDERSFIELD

QUEENSGATE
HUDDERSFIELD HD1 3DH

t: 01484 473969 **f:** 01484 472765
e: admissionsandrecords@hud.ac.uk

// www.hud.ac.uk

C741 BSc Medical Biochemistry

Duration: 3FT/4SW Hon

Entry Requirements: *GCE:* 200-280. *SQAH:* BBB. *IB:* 26.

K84 KINGSTON UNIVERSITY

STUDENT INFORMATION & ADVICE CENTRE
COOPER HOUSE
40-46 SURBITON ROAD
KINGSTON UPON THAMES KT1 2HX

t: 020 8547 7053 **f:** 020 8547 7080
e: aps@kingston.ac.uk

// www.kingston.ac.uk

CC16 BSc Biology and Sports Science

Duration: 3FT Hon

Entry Requirements: *GCE:* 200-280.

CCC6 BSc Biology and Sports Science

Duration: 4SW Hon

Entry Requirements: *GCE:* 200-280.

CC1Q BSc Human Biology and Sports Science

Duration: 4SW Hon

Entry Requirements: *GCE:* 200-280.

C741 BSc Medical Biochemistry

Duration: 4SW Hon

Entry Requirements: *GCE:* 280.

C744 BSc Medical Biochemistry (International only)

Duration: 4FT Hon

Entry Requirements: *GCE:* 40.

L14 LANCASTER UNIVERSITY

THE UNIVERSITY
LANCASTER
LANCASHIRE LA1 4YW

t: 01524 592029 **f:** 01524 846243
e: ugadmissions@lancaster.ac.uk

// www.lancs.ac.uk

BC79 BSc Biochemistry with Biomedicine

Duration: 3FT Hon

Entry Requirements: *GCE:* BBB. *SQAH:* BBBBB. *SQAAH:* BBB. *IB:* 29.

C1C7 BSc Cell Biology with Biomedicine

Duration: 3FT Hon

Entry Requirements: *GCE:* BBB. *SQAH:* BBBBB. *SQAAH:* BBB. *IB:* 29.

L23 UNIVERSITY OF LEEDS

THE UNIVERSITY OF LEEDS
LEEDS LS2 9JT

t: 0113 343 3999
e: admissions@adm.leeds.ac.uk

// www.leeds.ac.uk

C741 BSc Medical Biochemistry

Duration: 3FT/4SW Hon

Entry Requirements: *GCE:* AAB-BBB. *IB:* 32.

BC16 BSc Sports Science & Physiology

Duration: 3FT/4FT Hon

Entry Requirements: *GCE:* ABB-BBB. *IB:* 32.

M20 THE UNIVERSITY OF MANCHESTER

OXFORD ROAD
MANCHESTER M13 9PL

t: 0161 275 2077 f: 0161 275 2106
e: ug-admissions@manchester.ac.uk

// www.manchester.ac.uk

C724 BSc Medical Biochemistry

Duration: 3FT Hon

Entry Requirements: *GCE:* AAB-BBB. *SQAH:* AAAAB-AABBB. *SQAAH:* AAB-BBB. *IB:* 35. *BTEC ND:* DDM.

C741 BSc Medical Biochemistry with Industrial/Professional Experience

Duration: 4FT Hon

Entry Requirements: *GCE:* AAB-BBB. *SQAH:* AAAAB-AABBB. *SQAAH:* AAB-BBB. *IB:* 35. *BTEC ND:* DDM.

M40 THE MANCHESTER METROPOLITAN UNIVERSITY

ADMISSIONS OFFICE
ALL SAINTS (GMS)
ALL SAINTS
MANCHESTER M15 6BH

t: 0161 247 2000

// www.mmu.ac.uk

CX11 BA/BSc Biology/Teaching English as a Foreign Language

Duration: 3FT Hon

Entry Requirements: *GCE:* 220. *IB:* 26.

N84 THE UNIVERSITY OF NOTTINGHAM

THE ADMISSIONS OFFICE
THE UNIVERSITY OF NOTTINGHAM
UNIVERSITY PARK
NOTTINGHAM NG7 2RD

t: 0115 951 5151 f: 0115 951 4668

// www.nottingham.ac.uk

C741 BSc Biochemistry and Molecular Medicine

Duration: 3FT Hon

Entry Requirements: Interview required.

R12 THE UNIVERSITY OF READING

THE UNIVERSITY OF READING
PO BOX 217
READING RG6 6AH

t: 0118 378 8619 f: 0118 378 8924
e: student.recruitment@reading.ac.uk

// www.reading.ac.uk

C741 BSc Biomedical Sciences

Duration: 3FT Hon

Entry Requirements: *GCE:* 300.

R72 ROYAL HOLLOWAY, UNIVERSITY OF LONDON

ROYAL HOLLOWAY, UNIVERSITY OF LONDON
EGHAM
SURREY TW20 0EX

t: 01784 434455 f: 01784 473662
e: Admissions@rhul.ac.uk

// www.rhul.ac.uk

C741 BSc Medical Biochemistry

Duration: 3FT Hon

Entry Requirements: *GCE:* 300-320. *IB:* 34. *BTEC ND:* DDD.

S75 THE UNIVERSITY OF STIRLING

STIRLING FK9 4LA

t: 01786 467044 f: 01786 466800
e: admissions@stir.ac.uk

// www.stir.ac.uk

CX11 BSc Biology and Professional Education

Duration: 4FT Hon

Entry Requirements: *GCE:* CCD. *SQAH:* BBCC. *SQAAH:* AAA-CCC. *BTEC ND:* MMM.

S78 THE UNIVERSITY OF STRATHCLYDE

GLASGOW G1 1XQ

t: 0141 552 4400 f: 0141 552 0775

// www.strath.ac.uk

C1XC BSc Bioscience with Teaching

Duration: 4FT Hon

Entry Requirements: *GCE:* BBC. *SQAH:* BBBC.

S90 UNIVERSITY OF SUSSEX

UNDERGRADUATE ADMISSIONS
SUSSEX HOUSE
UNIVERSITY OF SUSSEX
BRIGHTON BN1 9RH

t: 01273 678416 f: 01273 678545

e: ug.applicants@sussex.ac.uk

// www.sussex.ac.uk

C743 BSc Molecular Medicine (Sandwich) (4 years)

Duration: 4SW Hon

Entry Requirements: *GCE:* AAB-BBB. *SQAH:* AAABB-ABBBB. *BTEC ND:* DDM.

W75 UNIVERSITY OF WOLVERHAMPTON

ADMISSIONS UNIT
MX207, CAMP STREET
WOLVERHAMPTON
WEST MIDLANDS WV1 1AD

t: 01902 321000 f: 01902 321896

e: admissions@wlv.ac.uk

// www.wlv.ac.uk

BC19 BSc Human Physiology and Biomedical Science

Duration: 3FT Hon

Entry Requirements: *GCE:* 260-320. *IB:* 30.

BCC6 BSc Human Physiology and Sport & Exercise Science

Duration: 3FT Hon

Entry Requirements: *GCE:* 160-220. *IB:* 30.

BIOMECHANICS

B32 THE UNIVERSITY OF BIRMINGHAM

EDGBASTON
BIRMINGHAM B15 2TT

t: 0121 415 8900 f: 0121 414 7159

e: admissions@bham.ac.uk

// www.bham.ac.uk

BJ95 BMedSc Biomedical Materials Science

Duration: 3FT Hon

Entry Requirements: *GCE:* BBC. *SQAH:* AAAAA-ABBBB. *SQAAH:* BBC. *IB:* 30. *BTEC ND:* DMM.

B80 UNIVERSITY OF THE WEST OF ENGLAND, BRISTOL

FRENCHAY CAMPUS
COLDHARBOUR LANE
BRISTOL BS16 1QY

t: +44 (0)117 32 83333 f: +44 (0)117 32 82810

e: admissions@uwe.ac.uk

// www.uwe.ac.uk

C601 BSc Sports Biology

Duration: 3FT/4SW Hon

Entry Requirements: *GCE:* 240-300.

C606 BSc Sports Biomedicine

Duration: 3FT Hon

Entry Requirements: *GCE:* 80-120.

D65 UNIVERSITY OF DUNDEE

DUNDEE DD1 4HN

t: 01382 383838 f: 01382 388150

e: srs@dundee.ac.uk

//www.dundee.ac.uk/admissions/undergraduate

CB69 BSc Sports Biomedicine

Duration: 4FT Hon

Entry Requirements: *GCE:* CCC. *SQAH:* BBBB. *IB:* 28. *BTEC ND:* MMM.

I50 IMPERIAL COLLEGE LONDON

REGISTRY
SOUTH KENSINGTON CAMPUS
IMPERIAL COLLEGE LONDON
LONDON SW7 2AZ

t: 020 7589 5111 f: 020 7594 8004

// www.imperial.ac.uk

BH81 BEng Biomedical Engineering

Duration: 3FT Hon

Entry Requirements: *GCE:* AAB. *SQAAH:* AAB. *IB:* 37.

BJ95 MEng Biomaterials and Tissue Engineering
Duration: 4FT Hon

Entry Requirements: *GCE:* AAB. *SQAAH:* AAB. *IB:* 36.

S18 THE UNIVERSITY OF SHEFFIELD
9 NORTHUMBERLAND ROAD
SHEFFIELD S10 2TT
t: 0114 222 1255 f: 0114 222 8032
e: ask@sheffield.ac.uk
// www.sheffield.ac.uk

BJ89 BEng Biomaterial Science and Tissue Engineering (3 years)
Duration: 3FT Hon

Entry Requirements: *GCE:* BBC-BBcc. *SQAH:* ABBB. *SQAAH:* BB. *IB:* 30 *RTEC ND:* DDM. Interview required.

SPORTS PSYCHOLOGY

B80 UNIVERSITY OF THE WEST OF ENGLAND, BRISTOL
FRENCHAY CAMPUS
COLDHARBOUR LANE
BRISTOL BS16 1QY
t: +44 (0)117 32 83333 f: +44 (0)117 32 82810
e: admissions@uwe.ac.uk
// www.uwe.ac.uk

CC68 BSc Psychology and Sports Biology
Duration: 3FT/4SW Hon

Entry Requirements: *GCE:* 240-300.

C607 FdSc Sport Performance
Duration: 2FT Fdg

Entry Requirements: *GCE:* 100-140.

C10 CANTERBURY CHRIST CHURCH UNIVERSITY
NORTH HOLMES ROAD
CANTERBURY
KENT CT1 1QU
t: 01227 782900 f: 01227 782888
e: admissions@canterbury.ac.uk
// www.canterbury.ac.uk

CM89 BA Applied Criminology and Sport & Exercise Psychology
Duration: 3FT Hon

Entry Requirements: *GCE:* 200. *IB:* 24.

N1CB BA Entrepreneurship with Sport & Exercise Psychology
Duration: 3FT Hon

Entry Requirements: *GCE:* 200. *IB:* 24.

C7CV BA/BSc Biosciences with Sport & Exercise Psychology (with Foundation Year)
Duration: 4FT Hon

Entry Requirements: *IB:* 24.

TC78 BSc/BA Sport & Exercise Psychology and American Studies
Duration: 3FT Hon

Entry Requirements: *GCE:* 200. *IB:* 24.

CGW4 BSc/BA Sport & Exercise Psychology and Digital Media
Duration: 3FT Hon

Entry Requirements: *GCE:* 200. *IB:* 24.

CX83 BSc/BA Sport & Exercise Psychology and Early Childhood Studies
Duration: 3FT Hon

Entry Requirements: *GCE:* 200. *IB:* 24.

CL83 BSc/BA Sport & Exercise Psychology and Sociology & Social Science
Duration: 3FT Hon

Entry Requirements: *GCE:* 200. *IB:* 24.

CN88 BSc/BA Sport & Exercise Psychology and Tourism & Leisure Studies
Duration: 3FT Hon

Entry Requirements: *GCE:* 200. *IB:* 24.

C30 UNIVERSITY OF CENTRAL LANCASHIRE
PRESTON
LANCS PR1 2HE
t: 01772 201201 f: 01772 894954
e: uadmissions@uclan.ac.uk
// www.uclan.ac.uk

C8C6 BSc Sport Psychology
Duration: 3FT Hon

Entry Requirements: *GCE:* 240. *IB:* 30. *BTEC ND:* MMM. *OCR ND:* Distinction.

D39 UNIVERSITY OF DERBY

KEDLESTON ROAD
DERBY DE22 1GB

t: 08701 202330 f: 01332 597724
e: askadmissions@derby.ac.uk

// www.derby.ac.uk

CC6V BA Sports Studies and Sports Psychology

Duration: 3FT Hon

Entry Requirements: *Foundation:* Merit. *GCE:* 160-240. *IB:* 26.
BTEC NC: MM. *BTEC ND:* MPP.

CCPV BA/BSc Martial Arts and Sports Psychology

Duration: 3FT Hon

Entry Requirements: *Foundation:* Merit. *GCE:* 160-240. *IB:* 26.
BTEC NC: MM. *BTEC ND:* MMP.

E84 UNIVERSITY OF EXETER

LAVER BUILDING
NORTH PARK ROAD
EXETER
DEVON EX4 4QE

t: 01392 263855 f: 01392 263857/262479
e: admissions@exeter.ac.uk

// www.exeter.ac.uk/admissions

C8C6 BSc Psychology with Sport & Exercise Science

Duration: 3FT Hon

Entry Requirements: *GCE:* AAA-AAB. *BTEC ND:* DDD.

H72 THE UNIVERSITY OF HULL

THE UNIVERSITY OF HULL
COTTINGHAM ROAD
HULL HU6 7RX

t: 01482 466100 f: 01482 442290
e: admissions@hull.ac.uk

// www.hull.ac.uk

C8C6 BSc Psychology with Sports Science

Duration: 3FT Hon

Entry Requirements: *GCE:* BBC. *IB:* 28. *BTEC NC:* DD. *BTEC ND:* DMM.

L27 LEEDS METROPOLITAN UNIVERSITY

COURSE ENQUIRIES OFFICE
CIVIC QUARTER
LEEDS LS1 3HE

t: 0113 81 23113 f: 0113 81 23129
e: course-enquiries@leedsmet.ac.uk

// www.leedsmet.ac.uk

C8C6 BSc Psychology with Sport & Exercise

Duration: 3FT Hon

Entry Requirements: *GCE:* 240. *IB:* 24. *BTEC NC:* DD. *BTEC ND:* MMM. *OCR ND:* Distinction.

L68 LONDON METROPOLITAN UNIVERSITY

166-220 HOLLOWAY ROAD
LONDON N7 8DB

t: 020 7133 4200
e: admissions@londonmet.ac.uk

// www.londonmet.ac.uk

CC68 BSc Sports Psychology & Peformance

Duration: 3FT/4SW Hon

Entry Requirements: *GCE:* 160. *IB:* 28.

N37 UNIVERSITY OF WALES, NEWPORT

CAERLEON CAMPUS
PO BOX 101
NEWPORT
SOUTH WALES NP18 3YH

t: 01633 432030 f: 01633 432850
e: admissions@newport.ac.uk

// www.newport.ac.uk

C6C8 BSc Sports Studies with Psychology

Duration: 3FT Hon

Entry Requirements: *GCE:* 280. *IB:* 24. Interview required.

PS